Vascular Neurosurgery in Environments with Limited Resources

Vascular Neurosurgery in Environments
with Limited Resources

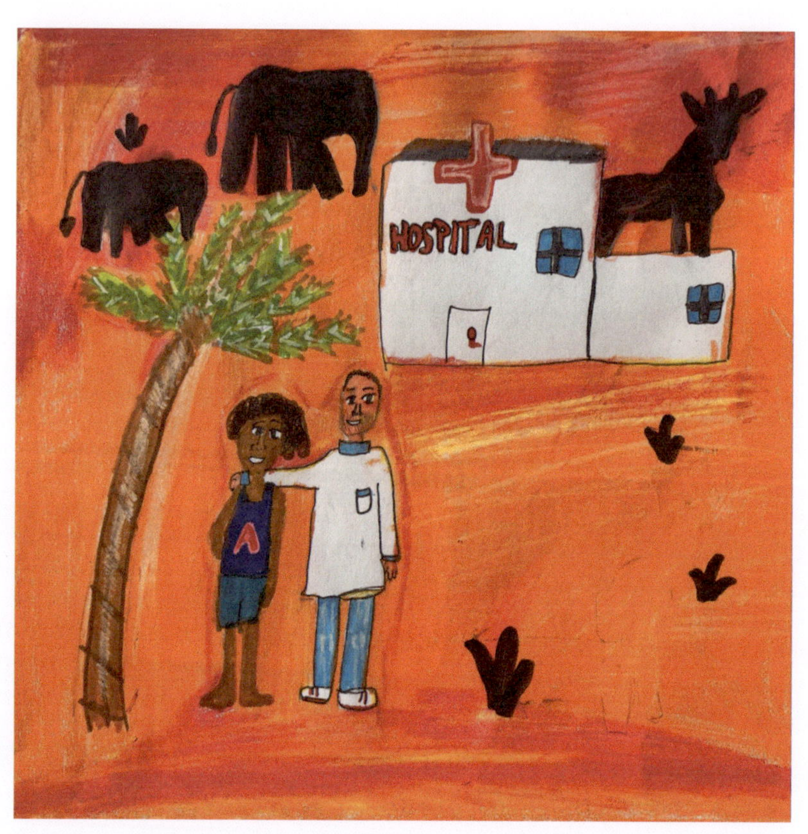

HOSPITAL
A

Athanasios K. Petridis
Homajoun Maslehaty

Vascular Neurosurgery in Environments with Limited Resources

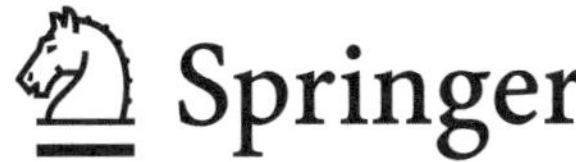 Springer

Athanasios K. Petridis
Neurosurgery
St. Luke's Hospital
Thessaloniki, Greece

Homajoun Maslehaty
Neurosurgery
St-Vinzenz-Hospital Dinslaken
Dinslaken, Germany

ISBN 978-3-031-59677-3   ISBN 978-3-031-59675-9   (eBook)
https://doi.org/10.1007/978-3-031-59675-9

This Springer imprint is published by the registered company Springer Nature Switzerland AG
The registered company address is: Gewerbestrasse 11, 6330 Cham, Switzerland

If disposing of this product, please recycle the paper.

Contents

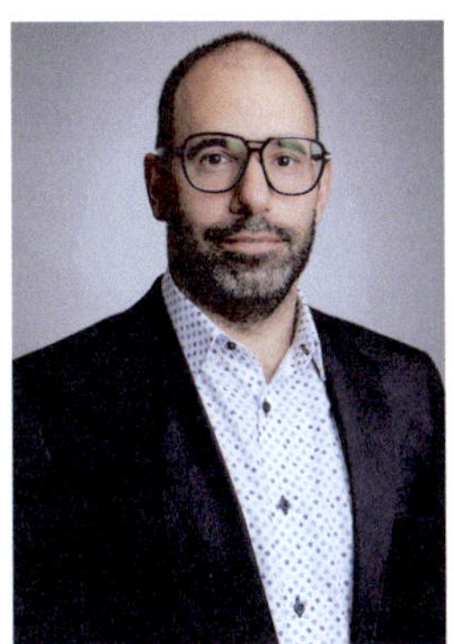

Athanasios K. Petridis is a 48-year-old professor of neurosurgery. He studied medicine at the University of Cologne, Germany, and became a doctor of medicine (virology) during his medical studies in Cologne. He started his residency in Kiel, Germany, with professor Mehdorn. During his residency, he completed a 3-year cellular and molecular neuroscience fellowship at the Memorial Sloan Kettering Cancer Center in New York City, USA. After finishing his residency in general neurosurgery in Kiel, he became an associate professor of neurosurgery in Kiel. He worked as an attending neurosurgeon and section director of oncological surgery as well as program director in spine neurosurgery for the AO Spine program in the neurosurgical department at SANA Klinikum, Duisburg, Germany. During this time, he got his first experience with vascular neurosurgery which he performed together with Prof. Scholz, the director of neurosurgery in Duisburg. After that and already having gained experience in the vascular field, he became director of vascular neurosurgery and full professor of neurosurgery at the Department of Neurosurgery, Heinrich Heine University, Duesseldorf. First, the cases were performed under the supervision of Prof. Steiger, and shortly, he took over the vascular department performing almost all vascular cases and publishing a big corpus on the vascular neurosurgery field. He is the neurosurgical program director of BRAIN Global. Together with Dr. Francis Fezeu, they initiated the first "on-site" fellowship in vascular neurosurgery at the Yaounde General Hospital, Yaounde, Cameroon. This fellowship has been completed, and two neurosurgeons are trained during 2 years in vascular neurosurgery. Another fellowship has been already started in MUHAS University, Dar es Salaam, Tanzania. More countries are in the waiting list. His vision is to train at least two neurosurgeons in vascular neurosurgery in every country of sub-Saharan Africa. Apart from being a vascular neurosurgeon, Prof. Petridis is a bachelor of theology and is also interested in philosophy and history. He is teaching "ethics in neurosurgery" at the Institute for History, Theory and Ethics in Medicine, Heinrich Heine University, Duesseldorf, Germany. Apart from the abovementioned professors whom he considers his teachers, he also stresses out the role of Dr. Harald Barth as one of his mentors. Prof. Petridis is a passionate diver and has been diving almost all over the earth, from wreck diving in Chuuk Lagoon to coral reefs in the north Forgotten Islands and snorkeling with whales in Tonga. He is an ambitious teacher of neurosurgery and a students' favorite as his students' evaluations show. At last but for sure very far from least, he is the father of Konstantinos, a handsome and young student of theology.

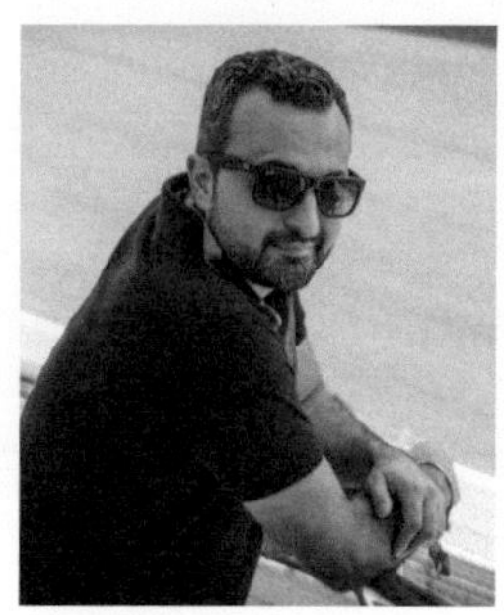

Homajoun Maslehaty is a distinguished neurosurgeon, educated at the University of Hamburg, where he earned his doctor of medicine title. He commenced his specialization training at the University Hospital Kiel and later served as a specialist at the University Hospital Essen.

He has made significant contributions to neurosurgery through a prolific array of scholarly works, including numerous scientific publications, book chapters, and lectures on neurovascular diseases. His academic achievements led to an appointment as an associate professor after completing his habilitation on neurovascular diseases at the University Hospital Essen.

As a senior physician and managing senior physician at Nordstadtklinikum Hannover, he further honed his expertise. In 2020, he assumed leadership as the head of the Department for Neurosurgery and Spine Surgery in Dinslaken, showcasing adept leadership in the medical field.

Abbreviations

A1	Anterior cerebral artery, pre-communicant segment
A2	Anterior cerebral artery, post-communicant segment
AcomA	Anterior communicans artery
aSAH	Aneurysmal subarachnoid hemorrhage
AVM	Arteriovenous malformation
C3-7	Cervical spinal cord vertebrae C3-7
CCA	Carotid communis artery
CSF	Cerebrospinal fluid
CT	Computed tomography
CTA	Computed tomographic angiography
DSA	Digital subtraction angiography
ECA	External carotid artery
EVD	External ventricular drainage
FDA	Food and Drug Administration
GCS	Glasgow Coma Scale
GOS	Glasgow Outcome Scale
IA	Intracranial aneurysm
ICA	Internal carotid artery
ICG	Indocyanine green
ICU	Intensive care unit
M1	Medial cerebral artery segment M1
M2	Medial cerebral artery segment M2
M3	Medial cerebral artery segment M3
M4	Medial cerebral artery segment M4
MCA	Medial cerebral artery
MRA	Magnetic resonance angiography
MRI	Magnetic resonance imaging
PCA	Posterior cerebral artery
PcomA	Posterior communicans artery
SAH	Subarachnoid hemorrhage
SSS	Superior sagittal sinus
STA	Superficial temporal artery
TIA	Transitoric ischemic attack
UIA	Unruptured intracranial aneurysm
WFNS	World Federation of Neurological Societies
WHO	World Health Organization

Introduction 1

Vascular neurosurgery undeniably stands as one of the most demanding disciplines within the field of medicine. Its focus lies in addressing disorders of the central nervous system stemming from vascular causes. Often, these conditions manifest as life-threatening states, demanding an intricate comprehension of neuroanatomical structures, alongside an exceptional level of precision and technique in executing procedures. However, the challenges of vascular neurosurgery extend beyond medical expertise. It necessitates sophisticated diagnostic equipment, a well-coordinated neurosurgical team and top-tier medical infrastructure. These are factors that are predominantly accessible in the Western world. In contrast, limited resources in developing countries result in significant impediments to medical access, diagnostics, and economic aspects.

Vascular neurosurgery primarily deals with conditions of the brain and spinal cord attributed to vascular issues. This encompasses, i.e., intracranial aneurysms, arteriovenous and cavernous malformations, and vascular stenoses. These ailments can trigger severe neurological symptoms and even become life-threatening if not promptly addressed. Vascular neurosurgery offers an avenue to substantially enhance the lives and well-being of afflicted patients, as it corrects vascular anomalies and restores normal blood flow.

The technical challenge of vascular neurosurgery lies in the imperative for procedures to be exceedingly precise and minimally invasive, so as not to harm surrounding healthy tissue. This necessitates sophisticated microsurgical techniques and an in-depth understanding of the intricate anatomy of the brain. This presents an immense technical challenge, given that the slightest oversight can lead to serious complications.

Crucially, diagnostic imaging plays a pivotal role in vascular neurosurgery. High-resolution imaging techniques like magnetic resonance imaging (MRI), computed tomography angiography (CTA), and digital subtraction angiography (DSA) are indispensable for identifying the precise cause of vascular issues and planning the most effective treatment approaches. These diagnostic procedures empower surgeons to visualize the exact location and size of aneurysms or arteriovenous malformations and accurately assess their vascular structures. Furthermore, they enable the measurement of blood flow in the brain or spinal cord, facilitating the evaluation of the severity of vascular stenosis or stroke.

In the Western world, these modern diagnostic capabilities are generally readily available and accessible. Patients can be diagnosed quickly and accurately, allowing for timely intervention. However, this is not the case everywhere in the world. In many developing countries, modern medical equipment and facilities are scarce, and patients have limited access to diagnostic procedures. This often results in vascular conditions being diagnosed only in advanced stages when treatment options are limited.

Another critical aspect of vascular neurosurgery is the neurosurgical team itself. Collaboration among neurosurgeons, neuroanesthesiologists, neurointensive care physicians, radiologists, and nursing staff is pivotal for the success of procedures. Each team member has specific roles and responsibilities, and precise coordination among all involved is indispensable to avoid complications and ensure optimal patient care. This necessitates not only excellent medical training but also intensive teamwork and communication.

In the Western world, highly specialized neurosurgical teams are widespread in large hospitals or university medical centers. These teams possess extensive experience in vascular neurosurgery and are familiar with the latest technologies and techniques. They have access to a wide range of resources to ensure the best possible care. In developing countries, however, such specialized teams are often scarce, and medical professionals often juggle multiple responsibilities simultaneously. This can compromise the quality of care and increase the risk of complications.

Furthermore, an essential factor in vascular neurosurgery is the quality of the medical infrastructure. Modern operating rooms, intensive care units, and postoperative care facilities are essential for ensuring successful treatment and patient recovery. In the Western world, such facilities are typically well-equipped and well-maintained. In many developing countries of the world, they are often scarce and underfunded. This can lead to shortages in care and jeopardize patient recovery.

Beyond medical challenges, there are also significant economic aspects influencing vascular neurosurgery in those countries. The costs of diagnostic procedures, surgeries, and postoperative care can be enormous, and many people lack the financial means to afford these treatments.

This often results in vascular conditions remaining untreated or being addressed only in advanced stages when the prognosis is poorer.

In this book, we share the experiences of vascular neurosurgical procedures in the countries of Tanzania and Cameroon gained by offering, organizing, and directing an "on-site" fellowship program together with the Brainglobal nonprofit organization. Beyond individual medical case examples, we delve into the broader context of vascular neurosurgery in these regions. We highlight the daily challenges faced by the dedicated physicians working there, including access to medical care for affected patients, the planning and execution of surgical procedures, as well as postoperative follow-up care. The aim is to share the experiences gained and to make the need for addressing this gap in medical care visible.

We will share insights into the unique challenges of cerebrovascular surgery in low-income countries with limited resources. We highlight the daily challenges faced by the dedicated physicians working there, emphasizing the need to train anesthesiologists and nurses.

Additionally, we will address the fear of craniotomy procedures among the local population, as well as the cost factor that can deter patients. Patient education is another crucial aspect of the on-site fellowship program, as it is essential to educate the population about the life-saving potential of seeking expert care when diagnosed with an aneurysm. Even a well-equipped cerebrovascular center must engage in patient outreach to fulfill its purpose.

We will present the results of the fellowship program, including follow-up examinations and the progress of local neurosurgeons. This will illuminate the learning curve of newly trained vascular neurosurgeons. These results have already been submitted in peer-reviewed journals, as scientific writing was an integral part of the fellowship, along with online and on-site educational lectures.

Current Treatment Standards of Cerebrovascular Diseases

We acknowledge that there exists a substantial discrepancy between the resources available in these advanced medical centers and those in regions with more limited access to advanced healthcare services, such as Central Africa. It is our hope that by illustrating the stark contrast between the two, especially concerning the management of intracranial aneurysms, we can foster a greater understanding of the challenges faced in underserved regions and the pressing need for global healthcare equity.

It's important to recognize that the treatment of cerebrovascular diseases is a complex and evolving field, and the specific diagnostic and therapeutic approaches can indeed vary from one medical center to another. Factors such as available technology, clinical expertise, and patient demographics all play a role in shaping the course of treatment. Therefore, while we provide a general overview, we also acknowledge the importance of tailoring treatments to individual patients' needs and the capabilities of each healthcare facility. And by training, we mean to work within the limitations we face. It is almost impossible to create a modern cerebrovascular facility and a developed-country fellowship program, when economical factors do not allow such an endeavor.

In conclusion, this chapter aims to showcase the impressive capabilities of modern neurosurgical and neuroradiological centers, emphasizing the critical importance of ensuring that such resources are accessible to underserved regions around the world. Achieving global healthcare equity is not only a noble aspiration but also a moral imperative, and we hope that this discussion serves as a reminder of the work that remains to be done in this vital area of health care.

2.1 Access to Diagnostic Imaging of the Central Nervous System

In regions like Japan and China in East Asia, there is a prevalent practice known as the "Brain Check-up" primarily due to the relatively high incidence of cerebrovascular diseases. These checkups often involve cranial MRI imaging. In contrast, in Europe and the United States, it has become increasingly common to perform CT or MRI scans of the neurocranium in response to various complaints, such as mild headaches or even after minor head traumas. We won't discuss further into whether this is solely done for forensic reasons to legally safeguard the treating physician at this point.

Consequently, this trend has led to the incidental discovery of intracranial neurovascular conditions more frequently. Conditions like incidental aneurysms, cavernomas, or arteriovenous malformations are being discovered by chance. This has opened up a new approach to the treatment of neurovascular conditions,

A. K. Petridis, H. Maslehaty, *Vascular Neurosurgery in Environments with Limited Resources*, https://doi.org/10.1007/978-3-031-59675-9_2

necessitating a careful consideration of the balance between the risks associated with treatment and the natural course of the pathology. From this arises the concept of preventive neurosurgery [1–4]. Overall, access to diagnostic measures in developed countries is often widespread and readily available. However, it's essential to consider the global disparities in healthcare access and resources, highlighting the need for equitable healthcare practices worldwide. Efforts to bridge these disparities, both in terms of diagnostics and treatment, are crucial to ensuring that everyone, regardless of their geographic location, has access to appropriate healthcare services.

2.2 Unruptured Intracranial Aneurysms

Unruptured intracranial aneurysms (UIAs) often come to light during various diagnostic investigations, frequently in response to symptoms such as headaches, dizziness, or a history of head traumas. Moreover, UIAs are commonly diagnosed in individuals with a hereditary or genetic predisposition, and they tend to be associated with specific medical conditions like polycystic kidney syndrome, fibromuscular dysplasia, Moya-Moya disease, Ehlers-Danlos syndrome type IV, and Marfan syndrome. The presence of these factors significantly contributes to the overall prevalence of intracranial aneurysm [5, 6].

The determination of which UIA should ultimately undergo treatment is a complex decision influenced by a multitude of factors. Various theories and approaches have been developed to assess the risk of rupture in UIAs, assisting clinicians in making decisions regarding medical interventions or continued observation with regular follow-up assessments.

On one hand, morphological parameters such as aneurysm size, configuration, location, and proximity to critical brain regions play a pivotal role in assessing the risk of rupture, providing invaluable insights into the potential danger posed by the aneurysm. However, it's worth noting that ongoing studies occasionally challenge the adequacy of this risk assessment methodology [3, 7].

Additionally, individual patient-specific risk factors come into play when determining the treatment plan. Factors such as high blood pressure, obesity, tobacco use, and other preexisting medical conditions collectively contribute to an increased risk of aneurysm rupture [8, 9].

In recent years, novel approaches have emerged with the aim of more accurately estimating the bleeding risk associated with intracranial aneurysms. These approaches delve into the composition of the aneurysm wall shear stress and meticulously analyze blood flow patterns within the vessels supplying the aneurysm and within the aneurysm sac itself, endothelial dysfunction, and inflammation [10–15a, b].

All these evolving methodologies aim to evaluate the individualized risk of bleeding in affected patients, ultimately helping clinicians make informed decisions about the necessity for treatment.

The decision-making process concerning the treatment of unruptured intracranial aneurysms remains a complex and dynamic challenge for both the treating physicians and the affected patients. Striking the right balance between the potential benefits and risks of intervention is paramount in providing optimal health care in these cases. As medical research and technology continue to advance, there is hope for more precise risk assessments and tailored treatment strategies, offering the prospect of improved patient care and outcomes in the future.

2.3 Ruptured Intracranial Aneurysms

The rupture of an intracranial aneurysm (IA) represents a pivotal and often life-altering event. It typically triggers a subarachnoid hemorrhage, which can manifest with or without an intracerebral hematoma. This critical condition demands immediate attention and intervention to mitigate potential devastating consequences.

The primary goal of surgical or interventional treatment in the acute phase is to promptly and effectively eliminate the source of bleeding, thereby preventing the occurrence of further hemorrhages. This step is crucial in averting the continued damage to brain tissue and the potential worsening of the patient's condition.

However, the management of a ruptured intracranial aneurysm extends well beyond the initial hemorrhage control. The true essence of therapy lies in addressing the numerous of secondary effects that result from the hemorrhage. These consequences can be complex and multifaceted, often involving critical aspects of neurological care.

One such complication is hydrocephalus, a condition characterized by an abnormal accumulation of cerebrospinal fluid in the brain's ventricles. Effective diagnosis and management of hydrocephalus are imperative to relieve intracranial pressure and improve patient outcomes.

Cerebral vasospasm represents another significant concern following a subarachnoid hemorrhage. This condition involves the constriction of blood vessels in the brain, which can lead to reduced blood flow and, ultimately, ischemia of brain tissue. Timely recognition and appropriate management of vasospasm are essential to reduce the risk of further neurological damage.

Furthermore, the aftermath of a ruptured intracranial aneurysm can involve complex systemic effects that extend beyond the brain. This includes the potential involvement of other vital organs, necessitating a comprehensive and multidisciplinary approach to care.

To provide the best possible outcomes for patients, a sophisticated and highly specialized intensive care setting is required. Such centers are equipped with state-of-the-art monitoring devices and staffed by skilled healthcare professionals who can deliver advanced medical interventions and act promptly.

It cannot be stressed out enough that the management of a ruptured intracranial aneurysm is a complex and multifaceted endeavor that encompasses more than just addressing the immediate bleeding source. It involves a comprehensive approach to diagnose, treat, and manage the various complications that may arise. Ultimately, the aim is to provide the highest level of care and support to patients in order to optimize their chances of recovery and overall well-being.

2.4 Diagnostics

2.4.1 Computed Tomography and Computed Tomography Angiography

Computed tomography (CT) is a valuable diagnostic imaging technique used in the evaluation of cerebrovascular diseases. It provides detailed cross-sectional images of the brain and blood vessels, aiding in the diagnosis and assessment of various cerebrovascular conditions, like ischemic stroke, subarachnoid, and intracerebral hemorrhages.

The significance of CTA, or computed tomography angiography, lies in its ability to rapidly and noninvasively identify the source of bleeding during critical situations (Fig. 2.1).

CTA provides a vital tool for healthcare professionals to swiftly and accurately pinpoint the location and characteristics of the aneurysm responsible for the hemorrhage. This information is pivotal in determining the most appropriate course of action, whether it involves surgical intervention or endovascular procedures to prevent further bleeding and manage the condition effectively.

Similarly, in cases of intracerebral hematoma, where bleeding occurs within the brain tissue itself, CTA offers a rapid and minimally invasive means of assessing the underlying cause. It allows medical teams to identify vascular abnormalities, such as an aneurysm or vascular malformation, that may have led to the hematoma. This diagnostic clarity is instrumental in guiding treatment decisions, ensuring that patients receive the most suitable and timely interventions.

The advantage of CTA is its ability to provide high-resolution images of the cerebral vasculature, allowing for detailed visualization of blood

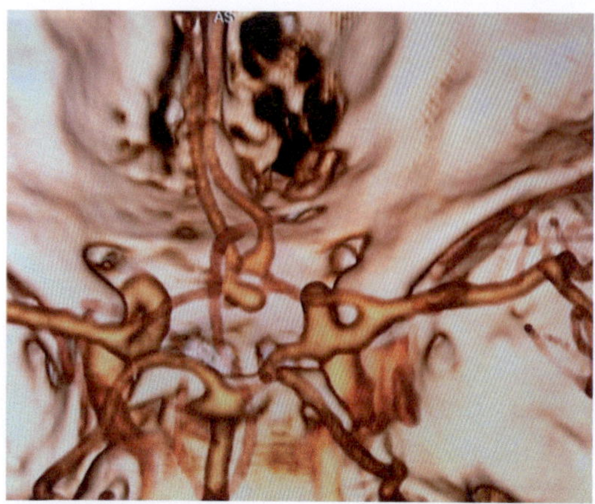

Fig. 2.1 CTA imaging example of a patient's case. Sometimes the available images are not enough to provide a full picture of the anatomy to the expert. It is possible to have a case where the patient comes to the hospital with only a CTA 3D reconstruction like the one showed in this image. How does the brain look like? How much available space will we have for the approach to the basal cisterns? How large are the ventricles? Is there any hydrocephalus? All these questions remain unanswered by the 3D CTA reconstruction. Be aware to check the available images by yourself (i.e., by the expert) and, in case information is lacking, to order new additional imaging (preferable cranial CT instead of MRI, which are affordable by the patients). For information on this specific case, see Chapter 7.3.1 and Fig. 7.20

vessels and potential abnormalities in 3D reconstructions. It offers a comprehensive view of the intracranial anatomy, aiding in the rapid diagnosis and subsequent planning of appropriate therapeutic strategies.

Furthermore, the noninvasive nature of CTA reduces the risk and discomfort associated with more invasive procedures, making it an invaluable tool, especially in emergency situations where time and patient well-being are paramount.

2.4.2 Magnetic Resonance Imaging and Magnetic Resonance Angiography

Magnetic resonance imaging (MRI) and magnetic resonance angiography (MRA) are diagnostic imaging techniques that are often not utilized in the acute setting when dealing with ruptured aneurysms. However, it assumes a pivotal role in the comprehensive diagnosis of incidental intracranial aneurysms, providing valuable insights into their anatomical characteristics, including their precise location, size, and configuration.

In the context of intracranial aneurysms, MRA offers a noninvasive and highly detailed view of the cerebral vasculature. Its ability to capture three-dimensional data allows for the creation of precise reconstructions, enabling healthcare professionals to visualize aneurysms in relation to their surrounding anatomical structures with exceptional clarity.

This imaging modality is particularly advantageous for assessing the spatial relationships between aneurysms and adjacent brain regions, blood vessels, and cranial nerves. Such detailed information is invaluable for surgical planning, as it aids in determining the optimal approach to treat or manage the aneurysm, minimizing the risk of damage to nearby structures and optimizing patient outcomes.

Moreover, MRA serves as a valuable tool for monitoring the progression of intracranial aneurysms over time. This is especially relevant for patients with known incidental aneurysms who require ongoing surveillance. Regular MRA scans can help track changes in aneurysm size and morphology, facilitating timely intervention if warranted.

While MRA does not play a primary role in the immediate management of ruptured aneurysms, its significance in the diagnosis, characterization, and long-term monitoring of incidental intracranial aneurysms cannot be overstated. It represents a noninvasive and highly informative means of understanding the complexities of these vascular anomalies, ultimately contributing to more informed medical decision-making and improved patient care.

2.4.3 Digital Subtraction Angiography

Digital subtraction angiography (DSA) remains the cornerstone of aneurysm diagnostics when it comes to assessing the brain's vascular system. It stands as the gold standard due to its unparalleled ability to provide precise information about the aneurysm's characteristics, including its configuration, location within the brain, and its relationship with adjacent arteries and veins. This level of detail is essential for accurate diagnosis and treatment planning.

The advent of three-dimensional rotational angiography has revolutionized the field of intracranial vascular imaging. This advanced imaging technique offers exceptionally high-resolution representations of the intricate network of blood vessels within the brain. As a result, clinicians can gain an even deeper understanding of the complex vascular architecture, allowing for more precise localization and assessment of aneurysms.

One of the remarkable aspects of this technology is its increasing accessibility and adoption. The continuous advancements in medical imaging technology, coupled with the widespread availability of three-dimensional rotational angiography, have democratized the diagnosis of intracranial aneurysms. It is no longer confined to specialized centers but is now widely accessible in medical facilities across the globe.

This expanded accessibility means that patients have greater access to early diagnosis and timely intervention, enhancing the overall quality of care for those at risk of or affected by intracranial aneurysms. As technology continues to advance, the field of aneurysm diagnostics and treatment is poised to make even more significant strides in patient care and outcomes.

2.5 Treatment of Intracranial Aneurysms

The treatment of intracranial aneurysms is a critical aspect of neurosurgery and vascular medicine, involving complex decisions that impact patients' lives profoundly. The primary goal of aneurysm therapy is to prevent the potentially devastating consequences of aneurysm rupture, such as subarachnoid hemorrhage, which can lead to severe disability or even death.

One approach to treating these aneurysms is through open microsurgical techniques. These procedures involve delicate and precise surgical interventions, often requiring a craniotomy to access the aneurysm directly. Microsurgical techniques have been refined over the years, with advancements in imaging, instrumentation, and surgical skills, making them a viable and effective option for many patients.

On the other hand, there are endovascular treatment options, such as coiling and stent-assisted coiling, which have gained popularity. These minimally invasive techniques involve navigating thin catheters through the vascular system to reach the aneurysm site, where coils or stents are deployed to seal off the aneurysm from the bloodstream. Endovascular procedures have the advantage of reduced surgical trauma, shorter recovery times, and potential applicability to patients who may not be suitable candidates for open surgery.

The choice between microsurgical and endovascular treatment depends on various factors, including the size and location of the aneurysm, the patient's overall health, and the experience, and expertise of the medical team. This decision-making process is dynamic, and advances in both surgical and endovascular techniques continue to shape the landscape of aneurysm therapy [16–18].

However, it's essential to recognize that this debate over treatment modalities is a luxury often unavailable in resource-limited settings, especially in developing countries. In these regions, where access to modern medical resources and highly specialized expertise may be scarce, the priority often becomes providing any form of treatment that can prevent aneurysm rupture and its potentially catastrophic consequences.

2.5.1 Endovascular Therapy for Intracranial Aneurysms

The endovascular treatment of intracranial aneurysms (IA) will only be briefly touched upon at this point. It would go beyond the scope of this book to delve into the individual therapeutic options. Instead, a brief overview will be provided to highlight the technically and instrumentally demanding method for the treatment of intracranial aneurysms [19].

Based on personal experiences and numerous conversations with local doctors and officials, we would like to emphasize at this point that endovascular therapy for IAs in Central Africa is associated with a variety of limitations and challenges due to limited resources and infrastructural obstacles.

Many parts of Central Africa face a significant shortage of specialized medical professionals, particularly neurosurgeons and neuroradiologists required for endovascular procedures. There are few well-equipped medical facilities in Central Africa that can provide the necessary equipment and technology for endovascular procedures, such as angiography and aneurysm treatment. Even when medical facilities exist, they often may not have access to advanced imaging technology and specialized equipment required for the safe conduct of endovascular procedures. In remote areas of Central Africa, transportation to medical facilities can be challenging. Road infrastructure and transportation means are often inadequate, making it difficult to provide timely care to patients. The costs associated with endovascular procedures and the required equipment are typically high, especially when it comes to the regularly follow-up imaging and the not uncommon need for recurrent endovascular treatments in cases of recurrence or recanalization of the treated aneurysm. Many patients in Central Africa have limited access to health insurance or financial resources to finance such expensive procedures.

Successful treatment of intracranial aneurysms often requires long-term follow-up and rehabilitation to monitor and manage potential complications. In many parts of Central Africa, the availability of postoperative care facilities is limited.

Coiling

In 1991, Gugliemi first introduced detachable bare platinum coil devices. This is considered the birth of endovascular coiling [20, 21]. By introducing platinum coils endovascularly, thrombo-sis and compaction of the aneurysm are achieved, effectively cutting off blood circulation. Over the following years, this method gained global acceptance for the treatment of IAs.

Balloon-Assisted Coiling

Balloon-assisted coiling, initially introduced in cardiac literature and subsequently adapted for use in cerebrovascular cases, represents a technique employed to treat wide-neck intracranial aneurysms. During the procedure for coil placement, a pliable balloon is inflated within the parent vessel, creating a temporary constriction within the aneurysm's neck. This constriction enables precise coil positioning within the aneurysm, preventing it from protruding into the parent vessel. This approach proves particularly advantageous when dealing with ruptured aneurysms featuring challenging anatomical configurations that are not suitable for standalone coiling. Various specialized balloon types, including hypercompliant, round-shaped, and double lumen balloons, are chosen based on the specific clinical context [22, 23].

Stent-Assisted Coiling

However, it wasn't until late 2002 that the first stent was specifically designed for the treatment of intracranial aneurysms (IAs). This groundbreaking development was the Neuroform stent, which received a Humanitarian Device Exemption from the Food and Drug Administration (FDA). Stents, in conjunction with coils, have proven invaluable in managing wide-neck IAs that cannot be effectively treated with coils alone or in combination with balloon-assisted coiling.

Stent design can be categorized into two main types: open-cell and closed-cell, each possessing distinct physical attributes. Closed-cell stents are characterized by smaller open areas between the struts, while open-cell stents feature larger uncovered spaces. The primary objective behind employing a stent is to provide a supportive framework that safeguards the integrity of the parent vessel, enabling the coiling of wide-necked, giant, fusiform, and other complex IAs that are not amenable to coiling in isolation.

Various stent configurations have been developed to achieve this purpose, including the R-stent, L-stent, nonoverlapping-Y, virtual-Y, horizontal, kissing-Y, and crossing-Y models.

One of the principal limitations of simple coiling is the high recurrence rate of IAs. Hence, the supplementary use of stents alongside coils aims to reduce this recurrence risk. More recently, novel endovascular devices have gained approval for the specific treatment of bifurcation IAs with wide necks. Notable among these devices are the pCONus1 and pCONus2, which are stent-like self-expanding nitinol implants with four to six distal petals that allow for coiling of the aneurysmal sac. Another innovation is the PulseRider, a self-expanding nitinol implant with a frame configuration that conforms to the vessel walls. These devices were engineered with the specific goal of preserving the patency of the vessel lumen and hemodynamic flow through the parent vessel bifurcation while minimizing exposed metal to facilitate endothelialization.

Excitingly, there are emerging devices such as the pCANvas, pCONUSTM, eClipsTM, and Comaneci. While comprehensive institutional data are still needed, recent meta-analyses have demonstrated high rates of technical success and acceptably low rates of morbidity and mortality in the use of these devices [24–27].

Double Microcatheter Technique

The double microcatheter technique provides an alternative approach for treating complex intracranial aneurysms (IAs) that present challenges for simple coiling. These challenges may include wide-neck aneurysm morphology or the presence of critical vessels branching from the aneurysm's base. This innovative technique involves the establishment of a stable coil framework by employing two coils that mutually support each other.

Before the coiling procedure begins, two microcatheters are strategically placed within both the proximal and distal regions of the IA dome. The initial coil is carefully positioned in the proximal section to create a supportive frame, while the subsequent coils are deployed through the distal microcatheter. This coil framework remains in place throughout the procedure until the aneurysm is adequately packed to satisfaction [28–32].

Flow Diverters

With the advancement of computational fluid dynamics and enhancements in imaging technologies in recent decades, there has been a growing focus on the design of medical devices. Flow diverters represent a new generation of neuroendovascular devices characterized by highly flexible tubular structures with mesh patterns, resembling stents in terms of engineering design. A significant distinction is that the mesh in flow diverters is less porous compared to typical stents. Consequently, the primary emphasis in the manufacturing design of flow diverters has shifted from solid mechanics to fluid mechanics.

The fundamental objective of a flow diverter is to redirect blood flow away from IA by placing a mesh structure, akin to a stent, at the neck of the IA along the parent artery. By decoupling blood flow between the parent artery and the aneurysmal sac, a flow diverter can induce blood stasis within the IA, promoting the formation of thrombus inside the aneurysm. Over time, the IA gradually undergoes thrombosis and regression, while the device serves as a scaffold for the development of endothelial tissue across the IA neck. This process results in the remodeling of the parent vessel and eventual resolution of the IA.

Flow diverters are designed for use in anatomical scenarios where standard coil-based treatments become challenging. Therefore, they are well-suited for wide-necked, giant, or fusiform IAs, offering a promising solution for these complex cases [33, 34].

2.5.2 Surgical Procedures for Intracranial Aneurysm Repair

Indeed, the stark contrast between the resources available to vascular surgeons in developed countries and those in developing nations is striking. In developed countries, the armamentarium for vascular surgeons seems limitless, with an array of advanced tools and technologies at their disposal.

For instance, companies like Aesculap and Mizuho provide an extensive range of aneurysm clip appliers and clips in various shapes and sizes. This diversity ensures that surgeons have the right tools for practically any aneurysm configuration (Fig. 2.2, see websites of the companies). With the assistance of 3D printers, it's even possible to create life-sized models of a patient's

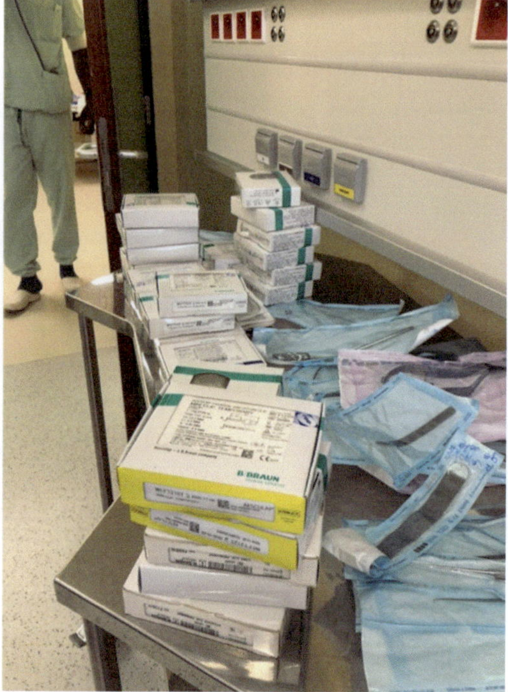

Fig. 2.2 Clips which have been ordered and delivered to the fellowship location by the expert himself. The expert has to know which clips he will possibly use and according to costs be aware that he cannot order any available clip, which the companies produce. Order clips which can be used for different aneurysms. If the expert has to choose between ordering a 90° fenestrated clip for aneurysms of the posterior wall of a vessel and a 90° non-fenestrated clip for aneurysms on the anterior wall of a vessel, the fenestrated clip should be ordered. The fenestrated clip can be used for both aneurysms and the non-fenestrated only for the anterior wall aneurysm. Order one clip, which serves as many purposes as possible. The expert uses clips and micro-instruments from B. Braun, since the company sold the equipment for a very low price, covering only the production costs. Charities from private sponsors and the gracious offer of B. Braun made it possible to equip the centers with all the instruments needed to efficiently perform cerebrovascular surgeries

brain vasculature, allowing surgeons to test different clips and order custom-made ones for exceptionally challenging cases.

In developed nations, the availability of these resources is often nearly instantaneous. Market competition in these countries ensures quick access to supplies. Even if a particular clip isn't in stock, replacements can typically be obtained within a matter of hours or, at most, within 12 h. Orders for surgical supplies are usually delivered within a day, regardless of the company you order from, thanks to efficient logistics and distribution networks.

Access to state-of-the-art equipment is another luxury. In countries like Greece or Germany, surgical suites are equipped with Zeiss and Leica microscopes, and with technicians who can quickly address any issues. In the rare event of a microscope malfunction, it can be swiftly replaced, and the technician can repair the damaged unit. However, the situation in Africa and other resource-constrained regions is different, where there may only be one microscope available, and it must function continuously. The availability of magnification for procedures becomes a crucial concern, and in some cases, surgeons resort to using loop glasses.

Intraoperative tools like indocyanine green videoangiography, which greatly assists in aneurysm clipping, are standard in developed countries but often unavailable in resource-poor settings. In Europe and the United States, hybrid operating rooms that incorporate angiosuites are increasingly common, enabling surgeons to promptly detect and correct misplaced aneurysms. Additionally, endoscopes are readily accessible for detailed inspection around aneurysms, and neuronavigation is available 24/7 for intricate procedures involving arteries like the pericallosal arteries, peripheral middle cerebral artery (MCA), or posterior cerebral artery (PCA) aneurysms.

The array of surgical instruments, from specialized knives to micro-scissors, is virtually limitless in developed nations. Retractors, retractor sets, and ergonomic surgical chairs with hand rests contribute to comfort and precision in the operating room. Suppliers of neurosurgical equipment showcase an extensive array of tools and technologies, all available for rapid delivery.

In conclusion, the gap in access to neurosurgical resources between developed and developing nations is a stark reminder of the disparities in health care around the world. While surgeons in developed countries benefit from cutting-edge technology and a vast array of resources, their counterparts in less fortunate regions often face significant challenges in providing optimal care to their patients. Closing this gap remains a critical global health challenge.

The prevalence of unruptured intracranial aneurysms in Europe and the United states is estimated to be around 1–3% of the adult population, although this can vary by country and region. Scandinavian countries have reported higher prevalence rates, possibly due to genetic factors and increased awareness of the condition. Prevalence tends to increase with age. Women generally have a higher risk of developing intracranial aneurysms. The availability of advanced medical imaging and increased awareness can lead to more frequent diagnoses in the United States and Europe [10, 16–18, 35–37].

However, Japan and Finland have some of the highest reported prevalences of intracranial aneurysms in the world, ranging from 3% to 7% of the population. The higher prevalence in Japan and Finland is possibly attributed to genetic factors. Additionally, these countries have well-established systems for early detection and treatment due to the higher prevalence [12, 38, 39].

On the other hand, the prevalence of intracranial aneurysms in Africa is challenging to determine. The reasons for this are multifaceted. Due to the lack of widespread cerebral imaging in various medical conditions such as headaches, dizziness, or head traumas, the rate of incidentally discovered but potentially life-threatening cerebrovascular diseases is relatively low. Furthermore, subarachnoid hemorrhage (SAH) can be difficult to diagnose as its symptoms can resemble those of other conditions. Misdiagnosis can occur when healthcare providers do not consider SAH as a potential cause of the symptoms. Accurate and timely diagnosis is crucial for appropriate treatment. Furthermore, the availability and access to neuroimaging, especially computed tomography (CT) scans or lumbar punctures, are limited, which is essential to confirm the presence of SAH. A lack of access to neuroimaging facilities or the failure to order these tests can lead to delayed or missed diagnoses. Moreover, due to the lack of systematic data collection and inadequate publications on this condition, it is challenging to estimate its prevalence accurately.

Tetinou et al. addressed this issue in an interesting publication. The authors conducted a search of published articles in various databases, including Medline, the World Health Organization (WHO) Global Health Library/Global Index Medicus, African Journals Online, and Google Scholar. They found a total of 33 articles from 13 African countries, listing 2289 patients with intracranial aneurysms up to the year 2020. This is an exceedingly small number considering the continent's population of approximately 1.5 billion. The authors conclude that the review suggests that the burden of cerebral aneurysms in Africa might be underestimated due to underreporting. They stress the need for further studies to better understand the epidemiological, clinical, and economic aspects of cerebral aneurysms in Africa at both the national and regional levels [40].

A. K. Petridis, H. Maslehaty, *Vascular Neurosurgery in Environments with Limited Resources*,
https://doi.org/10.1007/978-3-031-59675-9_3

Establishing Cerebrovascular Neurosurgical Programs in Central Africa: A Lifelong Decision to Take

4

Expertise in highly specialized fields of neurosurgery is often acquired beyond standard residency programs. Fellowships play a crucial role in mastering intricate areas like aneurysm surgery, the removal of arteriovenous malformations, obliteration of arteriovenous fistulas, and cerebral bypass procedures, among others. These complex surgeries demand a combination of structured training, access to basic equipment, and guidance from experienced vascular neurosurgeons. Ideally, the trainee should already be an experienced general neurosurgeon, before participating in a fellowship program at a dedicated center with an established vascular neurosurgery department. The key to successful training lies in the ability to perform a substantial number of cases during the fellowship, ensuring comprehensive and satisfactory training.

However, the situation differs significantly in many developing countries, such as Subsaharan Africa, when it comes to establishing highly specialized fields. To effectively address cerebrovascular cases, neurosurgeons in these regions require technical expertise, theoretical training in managing postsurgical cases in the ICU, and basic surgical equipment. Traveling abroad for 1 or 2 years for fellowship training is often challenging for these neurosurgeons due to the associated expenses and the critical need for their presence in their home departments. Even if they were to complete a fellowship in a well-equipped Western center, they may find it challenging to apply their skills back in their local environment, where technical equipment is often lacking.

In response to these challenges, we have initiated what can be described as a "reverse" fellowship or an "on-site" fellowship. An experienced vascular neurosurgeon from a well-equipped center travels to the location where the fellow should be trained, working within their local environment. This approach allows us to assess available resources, procure basic equipment cost-effectively, and adapt training to the local context. It is not sufficient to merely show a fellow how aneurysms are treated in the United States or Europe and expect them to encounter the same environment in Africa. It is more practical to have an expert on-site who can evaluate the possibilities and limitations of performing vascular neurosurgical procedures in a resource-constrained environment and then train the fellow accordingly.

We initiated this reverse fellowship approach and successfully completed it in Cameroon, with the program now ongoing in Tanzania. The results from the fellowship in Cameroon have been outstanding, with morbidity and mortality rates comparable to those in the Western world. This success is attributed to careful patient selection for surgery, with trainees operating under supervision on certain cases while experts handle others. We procured basic microsurgical equipment and aneurysm clip sets, which proved highly satisfactory. We also adapted to the delays in postsurgical CTA scans by prioritizing early extubation for clinical evaluations. In the absence of ICG angiography and microdoppler, we sharpened our observational skills, particularly our visual assessments of vascular structures.

Another significant aspect of the fellowship involves treating survivors of subarachnoid hemorrhages (SAH) in a region where a significant number of patients also suffer from HIV, resulting in vasculopathic vessels. Many aneurysms encountered were larger than those typically operated on in developed countries, surrounded by scar tissue and ruptured weeks to months earlier. Surgery on such cases is more challenging than what we are accustomed to, in the United States or Europe.

In this chapter, I (A. Petridis) aim to share my personal experience of working in Africa and my efforts to establish cerebrovascular surgery in this challenging environment (Fig. 4.1). My journey began when I was approached by the Brainglobal organization, which had a clear vision of creating an on-site fellowship program in Central African countries. However, resources were limited, including funding, which meant that we had to tailor a fellowship program to suit local circumstances. This entailed selecting only the most essential microsurgical instruments to master our surgeries (Fig. 4.2). The decision to participate in this program was one that I made without hesitation.

Now, having been involved in and directed two such fellowship programs in two different countries, with a third following shortly, I have no regrets, but I do have some words of caution for the next generation of trainers. First and foremost, Africa is not the place to train oneself. The cases encountered are exceptionally demanding, the equipment is rudimentary, and you often find yourself working in isolation. Be prepared to face cases that require a great deal of improvisation, creativity, and flexibility. We will delve into such cases later in this book. Issues may arise—perhaps the Mayfield head fixation is out of order, certain clip sizes and shapes are unavailable, the bipolar instrument is too short, or the suction force is too strong, to name just a few challenges. Moreover, the transition from the comfort of Europe to Africa, with rapid climate changes and the absence of air-conditioning in the operating room, can significantly affect concentration levels. If you cannot perform vascular neurosurgical procedures under such circumstances, disaster may be imminent.

Simply completing a dedicated vascular fellowship program in a Western country with 50+ cases and then packing your bags to demonstrate your skills to the African world is not enough. The "see one, do one, teach one" mentality does not apply in low-income countries. It's more like learning to swim in a pool and then suddenly finding yourself in open waters with 5–10-m waves.

Secondly, the cases will follow you. If a case fails due to equipment limitations, you must bear the consequences of your decision to proceed. The ability to decline a case because surgery is too risky is more prevalent in low-income countries. However, the patient's options if left untreated are also severely limited. You must find and provide an alternative for the patient. If trapping an aneurysm and performing a bypass is not feasible, postponing the case and equipping yourself with the necessary instruments is a better option. Always be aware of what can realistically be done; not everything is possible.

Thirdly, the fellows you train will become like your "stepchildren." Numerous questions will arise during your stay and even when you are absent. As the expert, you must take an active interest in your patients' follow-up. You may have patients in another country for whom you cannot be directly available, but you should still feel a direct sense of responsibility.

Last but not least, offering a fellowship means being committed to completing it and not abandoning the program midway, because it disrupts your daily work routine and surgical schedule back home. Agreeing to train neurosurgeons in Africa implies a commitment of at least 3 years of availability to them. It means being patient and prepared to teach in a fast-track fellowship program, where the learning curve accelerates. This is not about showcasting surgical skills; it's about performing surgery with a single aim—to enable local practitioners to independently perform such surgeries in the future, without the presence of an outside expert. Sometimes, guiding someone

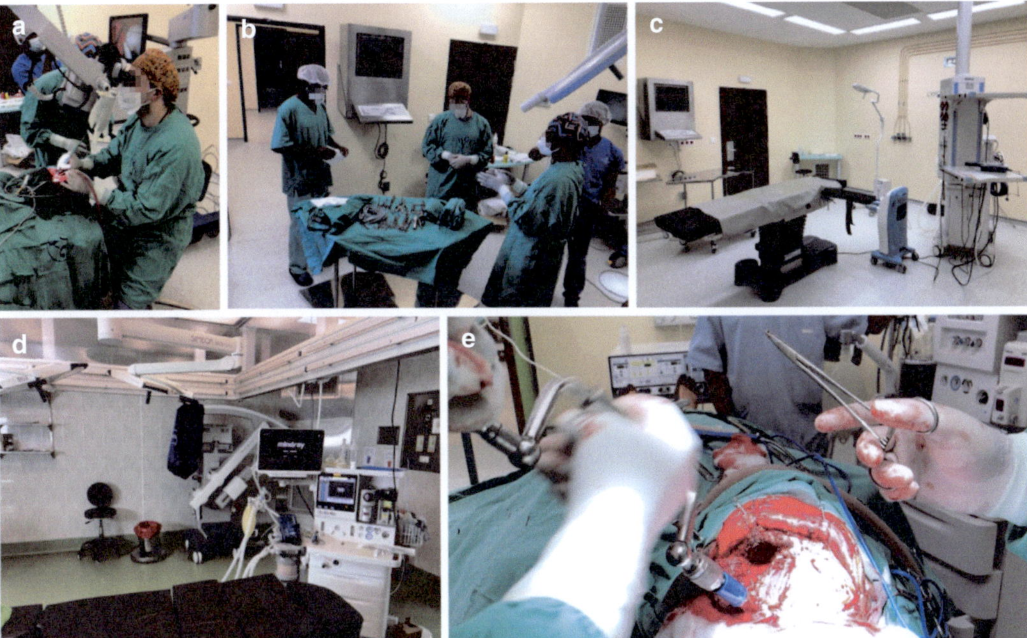

Fig. 4.1 A glimpse in the equipment of the local hospitals in Africa. From country to country, the equipment as well as the manpower can differ. It is always important to get a first impression of the operating rooms, the ICU, the available surgical instruments, and the experience of the trainees, scrub nurses, and anesthesiologists. (**a**) The operating microscope used in Cameroon, The magnification and handling of the microscope has to be checked before starting the first surgery. (**b**) The microsurgical instruments were controlled before surgery. We check the instruments before every surgery to be sure that we will not look around for instruments during the surgery. Language barrier can become a problem in explaining to the scrub nurse, which instrument has to be found during surgery. These problems are solved before they appear, by having the instruments on the operating table before cutting the skin. (**c**) The neurosurgical operating room in Yaounde, Cameroon. Coming to a new environment and planning to perform highly demanding surgeries needs a psychological and mental preparation of the vascular neurosurgeon. Where is the operating table located in the room, where is the position of the anesthesiologist, where the scrub nurse, and where the fellows are some of the essential facts you need to know in order to prepare yourself before surgery is started. After craniotomy, the environment does not play a crucial role anymore, and the focus is around the vessels, which are worldwide the same and familiar to the expert. It is like traveling through an unknown terrain to finally reach known territory. (**d**) Operating room of the neurosurgery department in Dar es Salam, Tanzania, Muhimbili University Hospital. There is a frame at the ceiling around the operating table (right upper corner to the left of the picture), which makes the move of the operating microscope close to the patient time-consuming. Therefore, the microscope is already moved into this area, before the skin is cut. This "frame" was something new to the expert, since it was not seen in other operating rooms before. The microscope is high, and the frame of the ceiling forces the team to push the Pentero 900 microscope very low in order to pass through the "frame." Space is needed for this reason, which is not available when patient and operating team are already in action. The microscope has to pass this obstacle before operation is started. (**e**) Handheld burr for burr holes. After that, the Gigly saw is used. A high-speed drill is available in both the fellowship locations, but in case two surgeries are planned or technical problems appear, there is no second drill in every location. So be aware that handheld devices have to be used too. In such cases, the craniotomy is performed by residents and fellows, who are very routined with the use of such devices

through the process of clipping a simple aneurysm demands far more patience than the most complex case you could perform yourself.

Additionally, it's important to recognize that even after the fellowship is completed, there will still be cases that are too complex for the newly trained vascular neurosurgeons to handle independently. For these cases, you must be prepared to provide lifelong support and assistance.

Expanding upon this journey, I want to emphasize the significance of collaboration and adapt-

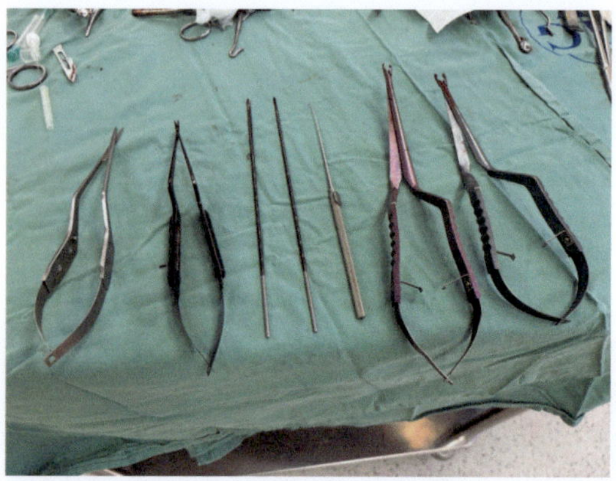

Fig. 4.2 Basic microsurgical equipment used by the cerebrovascular trainer. These are the basic micro-instruments, which are used by the cerebrovascular expert. From left to right, the instruments are micro-scissors with blunt tips, micro-scissors with sharp thin tips, two dissectors with different sizes, micro-hook, temporary clip applier of one size (which fits for deeper localized vessels, as well as vessels which are close to the surface, therefore choose a longer applier), and permanent clip applier. The clip appliers have to be tested for the specific clips. It is possible to have clips from one specific company and appliers from another (already available before the fellowship started), which will not fit on the clips. The best way to solve this problem is to let the expert be responsible for ordering the clips and the micro-instruments

ability in establishing cerebrovascular surgery in resource-limited regions like Central Africa. The challenges faced on this path are multifaceted, and each step requires careful consideration and innovative solutions.

In summary, my journey in establishing cerebrovascular surgery in Africa has been marked by dedication, adaptability, and a commitment to making a lasting impact. It is my hope that future trainers embarking on similar missions will find these insights valuable as they navigate the challenges and rewards of building neurosurgical expertise in resource-limited regions. Despite critics that this program is not in accordance to a western world fellowship, it is more worth than any hands-on cadaver course or a cerebrovascular symposium, where local neurosurgeons see cases, which have nothing in common with their reality. On the other hand, waiting for a sub-Saharan country to provide all the sources for a fellowship and then start it, will just leave the project in the planning stage, and it will never progress anywhere. Do not "talk the talk" but "walk the walk" as professor Juha Hernesniemi used to say.

5

Before delving into the details of this chapter, it is imperative to acknowledge that no matter how vivid our imaginations and expectations may be, the reality of working in low-income countries with their unique health systems will invariably exceed them. The circumstances one encounters in such environments are markedly different from those in well-equipped, high-resource settings. I (Petridis) will recount my experiences working in these challenging conditions and share valuable insights into establishing cerebrovascular surgery in Africa.

During my initial visit to Cameroon, we (Petridis and Francis Fezeu from Brainglobal) had planned to perform simple aneurysm clippings—a seemingly straightforward task. We had ordered some basic clips to carry out the procedures. However, upon arrival, we encountered unexpected challenges. The absence of a Mayfield head holder and the use of a bipolar instrument with an extremely short shaft, typically employed for coagulating skin, were among the obstacles we faced. The cases we tackled involved internal carotid artery (ICA) aneurysms and an arteriovenous fistula in a 5-year-old boy. Although we (me and the fellows) managed to complete these surgeries without complications, the notion of abandoning surgery altogether due to the local circumstances was a persistent thought throughout. Recognizing the need for improved equipment, we initiated the process of ordering essential instruments, such as a longer bipolar

device and micro-instruments like microdissectors, as a first step in our fellowship program. In Fig. 4.1, you can see the equipment used during the initial surgeries, the microscopes employed, and the operating theaters across different hospitals. Figure 4.2 displays the basic microsurgical equipment that was ordered and subsequently delivered for upcoming visits.

Our clip armamentarium is presented in Fig. 2.2. Notably, we did not have access to indocyanine green angiography and/or micro-Doppler for evaluating aneurysm occlusion and assessing the physiological perfusion of adjacent vessels. The specific challenges encountered during these surgeries and how we overcame them will be discussed in greater detail later in this book.

Another considerable challenge was the lack of functioning air-conditioning in the operating theater, leading to surgeries being performed in sweltering conditions with temperatures reaching up to 30 °C. Anesthesia posed yet another obstacle. A crash course in neuroanesthesia was conducted during the first surgery, covering critical aspects such as blood pressure control and the administration of mannitol to induce cerebral relaxation. During one of the surgeries, a moment of alarm occurred when the patient began to awaken mid-procedure, prompting a search for the anesthesiologist who had been called away to another theater. Consequently, we recognized the critical importance of training the anesthesia in our work, and an extensive focus was placed on

A. K. Petridis, H. Maslehaty, *Vascular Neurosurgery in Environments with Limited Resources*,
https://doi.org/10.1007/978-3-031-59675-9_5

this area. The entire team was educated about the gravity of aneurysm surgery and the necessity for unwavering concentration and focus. Before each subsequent surgery and after that, before every surgical procedure, discussions with the anesthesiology team were held. The fellows have now been trained to lead these conversations before every surgery too.

Assumptions about the team's awareness of the complexity of aneurysm surgery were deemed a mistake, and we understood the significance of comprehensive explanations. Many members of the team were entirely new to this type of surgery, and the expert's role extended to leading neuro-anesthesia, both before and during the surgery.

It's essential to avoid making assumptions in the realm of medicine, as assumptions can lead to catastrophic outcomes resulting from communication failures. This principle holds true not only in Africa but in every part of the world. It's important to be prepared for the possibility that the operating theater team may not be well-versed in the nuances of aneurysm surgery, and therefore, every aspect must be explained comprehensively. Every detail is new to some team members, and the expert surgeon must lead neuroanesthesia, instrument selection, and the choice of probable clips. Failing to address these matters before surgery can lead to confusion and inefficiencies in the operating room. We supplemented these efforts with lectures on the instrumentation used for aneurysm surgery, a practice we continued after the initial surgeries. Clarifying the importance of having someone in the surgical theater ready to provide clips immediately, instead of wasting time searching for them during surgery, was an integral part of our discussions.

Conversely, one of the most encouraging aspects of our work was the unwavering enthusiasm of the entire team to learn and listen. When issues were identified and solutions proposed, they were consistently well-received, and mistakes were not repeated frequently. It was remarkable to witness how quickly the team adapted to performing these complex surgeries exactly as discussed and taught. Following the completion of the fellowship, the level of anesthesia performance has reached an exceptional standard. Additionally, awake vascular surgeries have been successfully performed twice with satisfactory results. The team's enthusiasm for learning proved to be our most potent asset in aneurysm surgery in low-income countries. There is no shame in being inexperienced, as long as there is a willingness to discuss and rectify errors among open-minded individuals eager for change. We were privileged to work with a highly dedicated team that achieved a remarkable level of expertise, leading to near-zero disasters attributable to the team's capabilities. The exceptional efficiency demonstrated during the occlusion of a ruptured ICA aneurysm in just 29 min microscope-time by one of the fellows, with the inclusion of a proficient scrub nurse, reflects the team's outstanding competence. The patient's outcome was nothing short of excellent. The team's ability to learn, read, and self-educate, resulting in gradual case-by-case improvement, exceeded all expectations and contributed significantly to the remarkable efficiency they have attained.

Another critical aspect that demands consideration is the expert surgeon's health and safety. It is essential to be aware that a significant number of patients may be HIV-positive, necessitating extreme caution to avoid injuries that could expose the surgeon to infected blood, such as cut injuries or blood splattering onto the face. Malaria prevention measures must be taken during the stay in these regions and even upon returning home. However, it's important to note that malaria prophylaxis drugs, such as Malarone, can have adverse effects, including hallucinations and heart rhythm abnormalities (see Malarone and its adverse effects). Working under the influence of such medication is a challenge that surgeons must overcome. Additionally, skin infections, eye infections, and ear infections can become problematic, since not every pharmacy stocks antibiotic drops or antibiotics. Generally, safety concerns extend beyond the operating room to the streets, where walking alone can be a considerable risk. Even local doctors are cautious about the safety of foreign doctors navigating unfamiliar surroundings. Furthermore, consuming untreated water and non-boiled food is virtually guaranteed to lead to diarrhea in every instance. Surgeons may find themselves in a situation where they must perform complex aneurysm surgery while dealing with the side effects of malaria prophylaxis, an eye infection, and diarrhea simultaneously. Preparing for this worst-case scenario by organizing a personal pharmacy within your travel bag is advisable. It is essential to bear in mind that you will be performing intricate aneurysm surgery in an environment that can push your body and mind to their limits. This includes the realization that the personnel working with you, at least initially, may have little awareness of the nature of the surgery you are undertaking.

Patients with intracranial aneurysms or other vascular malformations were referred either by primary care physicians or other nationwide hospitals. Initially, these patients were examined by resident doctors and then presented to physicians within the vascular fellowship program. The patient's history, neurological status, and gathered findings, along with available radiological results, were discussed in an online meeting with the neurovascular expert surgeon. The case was deliberated upon, and a decision for surgical intervention was made. Patients were given a fixed appointment scheduled for the time when the expert surgeon planned to be in the country. They have to schedule a flight from other areas to get admitted to the hospital on the right time.

At this point, we would like to highlight the limited and often insufficient cerebral imaging, particularly by European standards. The preoperative high-resolution digital subtraction angiography, commonly used in Western countries, is almost never available.

The presurgical imaging examinations for diagnosing aneurysms typically involved CT or MR angiography. However, CTA and MRA imaging often exhibited low quality, lacking reconstruction, and having a thick slice thickness. This limitation hindered drawing conclusions about the aneurysm's anatomy. In certain instances, the precise origin of the aneurysm couldn't be identified. Specifically concerning A1-A2 junction aneurysms, determining the side (left or right) of the artery bearing the aneurysm was not feasible. Consequently, we were required to approach the aneurysm and clarify the surrounding anatomy exclusively during the intraoperative phase.

Figure 2.1 illustrates a case involving an HIV-positive patient with an A1-A2 junction aneurysm on the left side and an indication of vessel dilation at the origin of A2 on the right side. Our approach targeted the aneurysm from the right side during surgery to clarify the anatomical details. During the procedure, manipulation around the aneurysms was necessary, resulting in a controllable rupture occurring on both aneurysms. Notably, the A1-A2 junction aneurysm on the right side exhibited extensive thrombosis and was larger than anticipated.

Relying solely on CTA and MRA for preoperative imaging in aneurysm surgeries may create a potential risk due to the possibility of unexpected variations in aneurysm anatomy. Consequently, there remains a small margin of uncertainty regarding the actual anatomy of the aneurysm. While this doesn't invariably lead to disastrous outcomes, it underscores the importance of preparedness for thorough anatomical exploration during surgery to precisely locate the aneurysm neck. The surgeon cannot be entirely certain about approaching the aneurysm from the

© The Author(s), under exclusive license to Springer Nature Switzerland AG 2024
A. K. Petridis, H. Maslehaty, *Vascular Neurosurgery in Environments with Limited Resources*,
https://doi.org/10.1007/978-3-031-59675-9_6

side where the neck is situated. This emphasizes the need for caution and meticulous assessment intraoperatively to ensure accurate surgical navigation.

When approaching an aneurysm, the procedure involves freeing it by dissection and identifying its neck on the vessel from which it originates, which might even be situated on the opposite side. It's essential to note that most of the aneurysms we operate on have previously ruptured, rendering them unstable. This instability adds an extra layer of complexity to the surgical process.

Throughout this book, we will delve into specific cases where we'll illustrate and discuss the imaging quality associated with these aneurysms. In Fig. 6.1, several examples of the aneurysm clips that we utilize during our procedures are depicted, providing visual insight into the tools and techniques employed in our work.

Adding to the challenge, CTA or MRA stands as the sole diagnostic imaging modality available for arteriovenous fistulas and arteriovenous malformations. While these scans enable us to identify the nidus—the central region of abnormal vasculature—the intraoperative identification of feeding arteries and draining veins becomes imperative. The absence of DSA which provides precise data regarding feeding arteries necessitates our reliance on CTA and MRA. With these imaging modalities, we meticulously identify all vessels leading to the nidus and carefully dissect them during surgery. Nevertheless, the lack of exact data about feeding arteries compels us to perform temporary occlusions on vessels that remain uncertain in their role, whether as feeding arteries or draining veins (Fig. 6.2).

During our fellowship, we accomplished successful extractions of arteriovenous malformations (AVMs) in two patients. One patient presented with an AVM located in the lateral ventricle (Fig. 6.3), while the other had an AVM in the left frontal lobe near the midline (Fig. 6.4). In these instances, our approach involved dissecting

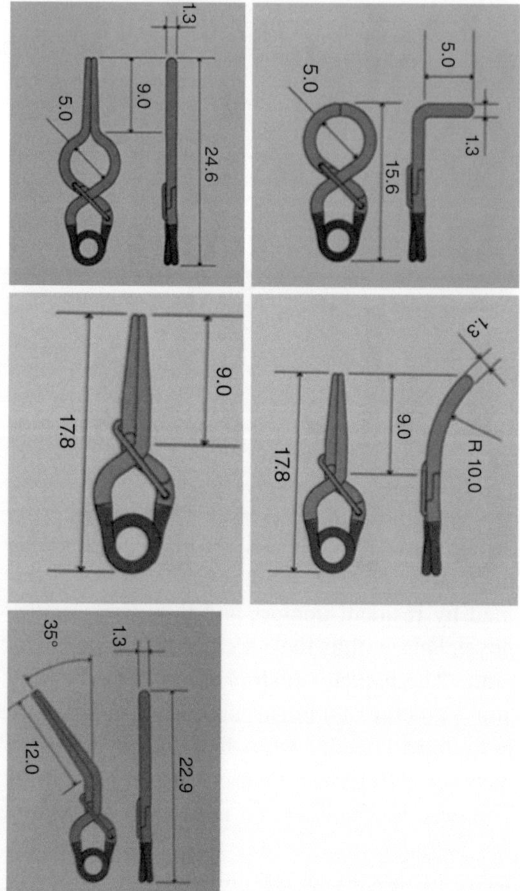

Fig. 6.1 Shapes of the clips in use. These are basically the shapes and sizes of the clips we use in the fellowships in order to hold costs low and still be efficient. The main company we work with is B. Braun. In some centers, there are clips from Mizuho already available, which are excellent too. The clips can be available though without the necessary clip applier, which can make the clip worthless (in many cases and after improvisation the clips can be still used but reapplication, clip removal, etc. with the wrong unfitting applier can bring the clip to snap and lead a catastrophic event). Check for the available clips means to check for the available appliers too

the nidus and promptly occluding all vessels, regardless of whether they were veins or arteries. This was feasible, since we had dissected the AVM entirely and could oversee the structure.

Despite the presence of angio-suites in the facilities in Cameroon, the absence of a dedi-

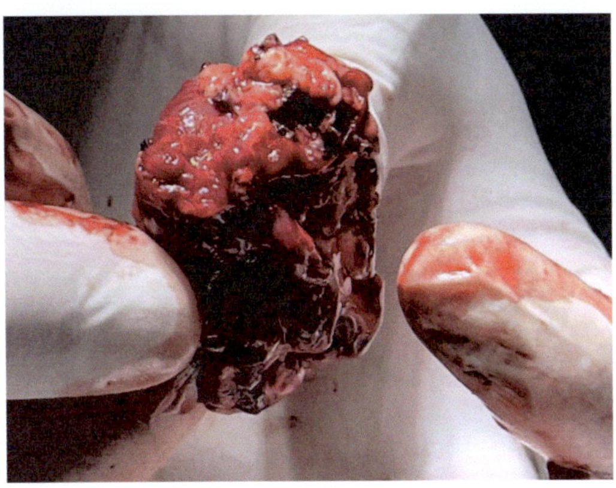

Fig. 6.2 A completely removed AVM of the precentral area. The preoperative imaging, which was available was a CTA, since DSA is in most cases not available

cated neuroradiologist capable of performing such angiographies remains a limitation. However, we anticipate future improvements in neuroimaging services to optimize care for neurovascular cases.

Regrettably, intraoperative imaging modalities like ICG videoangiography and micro-Doppler are unavailable to us. Therefore, in most cases, after clipping aneurysms, we resort to perforation to ensure complete occlusion and obtain a clearer view of the arteries proximal and distal to the aneurysms. Visual inspection of vessels before and after clipping remains the only method to control stenosis or arterial occlusion caused by a clip.

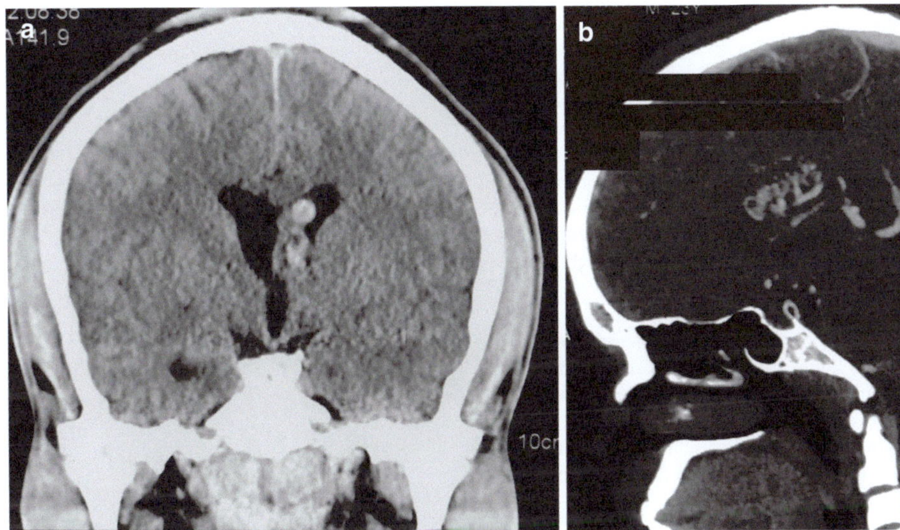

Fig. 6.3 AVM of the left lateral ventricle. This AVM bled multiple times. It was completely removed by the cerebrovascular expert during the on-site fellowship. Only the CTA was available for planning the surgery. DSA was not available and therefore information about feeding arteries and draining veins could only be guessed by the anatomy. In the present case, such a guess was not impossible even by a static CTA. The vessel which leads to the internal cerebral vein would be a vein. Vessels originating from the pericallosal arteries would be feeding arteries. Never the less some feeders can be missed without a DSA imaging, which forces the surgeon to dissect around the AVM with meticulous technique and stay away from the nidus, i.e., stay at the borders of the AVM and do not rupture vessels of the nidus, which would lead to a bleeding. During this case, which is descried in Chapter 7.7.1, dissection was easy, since the AVM was located exclusively in the lateral ventricle making the dissection around the nidus safe. Intraparenchymal cases can be more difficult to handle, especially when feeders are not identified in a preoperative DSA. (**a**) Coronal section. The AVM is located in the left lateral ventricle. (**b**) Sagittal section

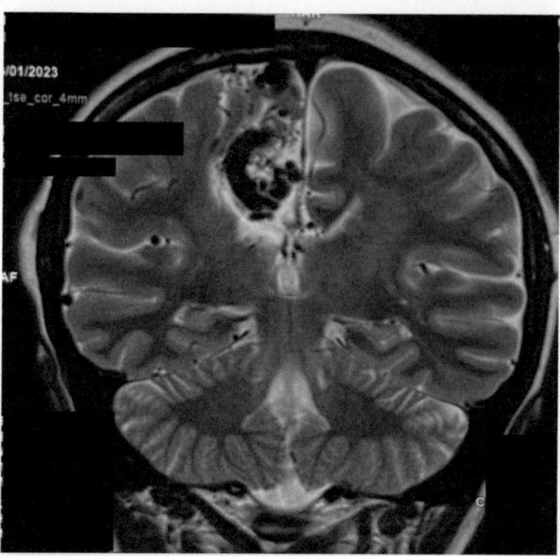

Fig. 6.4 Precentral AVM of the right side. This precentral AVM was removed completely with the only available preoperative imaging the MRA. Since dissection in such a critical area has to be very close to the nidus and the feeder location was not clearly identified through the lack of DSA, the risk of damaging the precentral cortex was high. We would not perform this surgery if the patient was neurologically intact. Since the patient had a hemiplegia for years and a bleeding of the AVM some years ago, we could perform the surgery with minimum risk of creating new neurological deficits, with the aim to prevent another bleeding (see also Chapter 7.7.2). Otherwise we would not proceed with surgery without DSA. Indications of such surgeries have to be carefully given and always keep in mind that preoperative planning is incomplete in low-income countries with limited resources. Efforts are done to have diagnostic DSA in the newly establishing cerebrovascular centers. This is economically affordable and in no comparison with expensive endovascular procedures. However, the information for the surgeon and for preoperative planning is of highest value

In this chapter, we aim to present selected intriguing cases. The detailed descriptions of these cases will highlight substantial differences and challenges in microsurgical neurovascular treatment, contrasting with the therapeutic standards of the Western world. We seek to demonstrate that even complex neurovascular procedures can be performed considering the resources and limitations prevalent in Central Africa. However, our collected experiences underscore a pressing need for significant enhancements in medical infrastructure, diagnostic imaging, therapy, and postoperative care, especially concerning neurovascular diseases. Improving these aspects is crucial for better safeguarding the health of affected patients.

We will illustrate the surgical technique and typical cases encountered during an on-site fellowship. We'll commence with the discussion of MCA (middle cerebral artery) aneurysms, ICA (internal carotid artery), and PcomA (posterior communicating artery), AcomA (anterior communicating artery), as well as pericallosal artery aneurysms.

One key factor distinguishing surgeries in African countries from those in Western nations is the typical larger size of aneurysms. These larger aneurysms often lead to symptomatic presentations, such as paralytic PcomA aneurysms. Additionally, many cases involve aneurysms that have ruptured months prior, resulting in the presence of scar tissue and thick arachnoid villi around the aneurysm.

Toward the chapter's conclusion, we will present cases of typical subarachnoid hemorrhage that appeared negative for aneurysms in CTA. Due to the lack of DSA, we were compelled to perform explorative neurosurgery. Among the four patients operated on in an exploratory manner, one case revealed a paraophthalmic aneurysm surrounded by a blood clot, which we subsequently clipped. However, in the remaining three cases, neither an aneurysm nor a bleeding source could be identified.

Every case starts with a talk about the planned surgery with the team, which consists of the anesthesiologist, the scrub nurse, and the fellows. The positioning and the equipment to be used are communicated to the team, and the functionality of the microscope, craniotome, and the rest of the equipment is checked by the expert and the fellows.

7.1 Treatment of Middle Cerebral Artery (MCA) Aneurysms

7.1.1 M2-M3 Bifurcation Aneurysm

The initial case we aim to illustrate involves the surgery for a ruptured left-sided M2-M3 bifurcation aneurysm in a 54-year-old female patient. The rupture occurred 6 weeks prior to the surgical intervention. Preoperatively, the patient did not display any neurological deficits and was admitted to the hospital 1 day before the scheduled surgery.

According to the findings of the CCT and CTA, the aneurysm could be identified. The presence of cerebral vasospasm seemed unlikely based on the findings, although a certain parenchymal hypodensity was discussed as a possible sign of parenchymal edema (Fig. 7.1).

The exclusion of vasospasm to the best extent possible is crucial before surgery. If vasospasms are present, surgery should be postponed, since they can worsen, due to unregulated suction that may inadvertently damage vessels, further exacerbating the vasospasm. Another reason to exclude vasospasm is the use of mannitol and hypotension during surgery (in order to have a relaxed brain) which would have a deleterious effect in a vasospastic brain.

The preoperative MRI of the brain revealed remnants of a frontal lobe hematoma (Fig. 7.2). Given the location of this aneurysm within the Sylvian fissure, coupled with its previous rupture, we anticipated the aneurysm to adhere to brain tissue. Additionally, we expected the arachnoid within the Sylvian fissure to be thickened and scarred.

After initiating an intubation anesthesia, the patient received 200 mL of 20% mannitol from the anesthesiologist, as instructed by the expert surgeon, while maintaining the blood pressure below 110 mmHg systolic. The patient's body was positioned in an anti-Trendelenburg orientation at 20°. Following the three-point fixation of the head (at 60° to the right and 25° of retroflexion) and sterilization, a craniotomy was per-

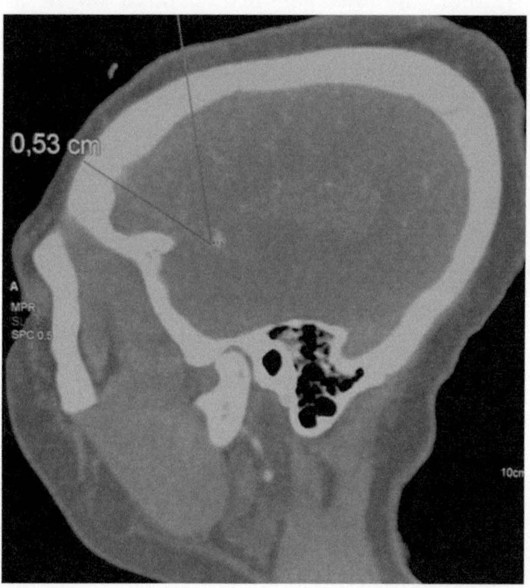

Fig. 7.1 M2-M3 bifurcation aneurysm. Sagittal CTA reconstruction of the M2-M3 aneurysm. The aneurysm was 5 mm in size. Problems which could appear are to find the aneurysm in the periphery. No neuronavigation can sometimes lead to search around the vessels and damage intact brain tissue. Keeping this in mind, we identified first which M2 was the artery of origin of the aneurysm and planned to dissect the artery from the M1-M2 bifurcation to the aneurysm. The Sylvian fissure has to be opened distally for about 3 cm. Figure 7.3 illustrates the surgery

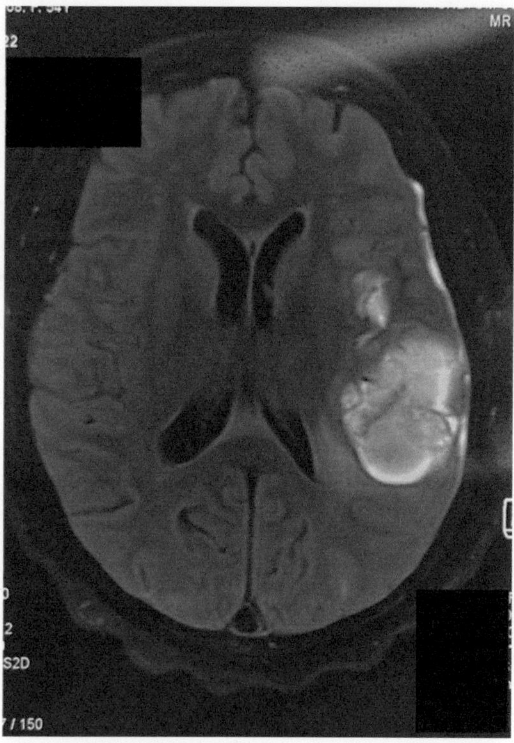

Fig. 7.2 The MRI of the ruptured M2-M3 aneurysm (see Fig. 7.1 too) shows the intraparenchymal bleeding, which was caused by the aneurysm. The aneurysm was ruptured 6 weeks ago, but from the MRI alone, there cannot be said for sure if another bleeding occurred in the meantime

formed using a handheld trephine and Gigli saw. Creating space in the edematous brain involved removing some hygroma from the bleeding cavity. Predominantly, precise dissection was necessary to access the aneurysm, and it was more logical to commence from the MCA M1-M2 bifurcation, following the superior branch to the M2-M3 bifurcation.

The Sylvian fissure was delicately opened by the fellow to ensure avoidance of damaging the veins within the fissure. Our aim was to preserve these veins intact, especially the larger ones, even if it meant sacrificing the smaller branches. Progressing along the superior trunk of the M2, sharp dissection was used to free the vessel while applying controlled tension with suction, employing the suction as a blunt dissector in the left hand and microscissors for precise dissection in the right hand. Tracing the M2 toward its M3 bifurcation allowed us to locate the aneurysm. Subsequently, the aneurysm was carefully dissected from the adjacent arteries of the M3 using blunt dissection. To alleviate tension on the aneurysm and prevent re-rupture during further dissection of the neck, the proximal M2 was temporarily clipped for approximately 2 min.

The arteries were gently maneuvered away from the aneurysm neck to create ample space for the application of a clip around the neck. A 7 mm slightly curved clip was utilized to occlude the aneurysm. Following the occlusion, the aneurysm dome was carefully dissected free, and the M3 arteries were identified and traced distally to ensure there was no stenosis or occlusion caused by the clip (refer to Fig. 7.3).

Immediately postsurgery, the patient was awakened to promptly assess for any signs of nerve palsies. Subsequently, she was transferred to the ICU where she received 2 L of fluids over the next 24 h, was allowed free oral liquids, and her blood pressure was maintained within physiological levels (i.e., 110–140 mmHg systolic). The following day, a postoperative CTA and CCT were conducted, revealing no remnants of the aneurysm and no signs of infarctions that would suggest occlusion of neighboring vessels (see Fig. 7.4).

7.1.2 M1-M2 Bifurcation Aneurysm with STA-M4 (Superior Temporal Artery: Middle Cerebral Artery) Bypass

A 43-year-old male patient, previously diagnosed with a subarachnoid hemorrhage 2 months ago, was admitted for the clipping of an MCA aneurysm located on the right side, which was identified as the source of his bleeding. Upon admission, he presented with no neurological deficits. A CCT scan conducted 2 months earlier revealed the presence of SAH, while the CTA pinpointed an MCA bifurcation (specifically the M2 superior trunk) aneurysm as the likely cause of the hemorrhage (Fig. 7.5). However, the CTA failed to clearly identify the neck and the origin of the artery associated with the aneurysm.

The decision to proceed with aneurysm clipping was made. In the event that the origin artery of the aneurysm would involve the M2 segment, we opted to prioritize the placement of an STA-M4 MCA bypass beforehand to ensure the artery remained unobstructed or, in the case of potential occlusion, to mitigate any issues before proceeding with the aneurysm clipping.

During the procedure, the patient's head was fixed at a position of 60° to the left and 30° in retroflexion. Administration of mannitol and maintenance of a systolic blood pressure below 110 mmHg were necessary to maintain brain relaxation. The STA (superficial temporal artery) was identified via palpation, and a 8 cm long arterial segment was dissected free and cut distally. A temporary clip was applied as close to the proximal site as feasible. The donor artery was meticulously dissected away from perivascular tissue, and the opening was shaped like a fishmouth (Fig. 7.6). The segment underwent an intraluminal rinse with a heparin solution. Notably, the patient did not receive any preoperative heparinization or anticoagulants of any kind. For detailed bypass techniques, we refer to the book "7 Bypasses" by Michael Lawton [41].

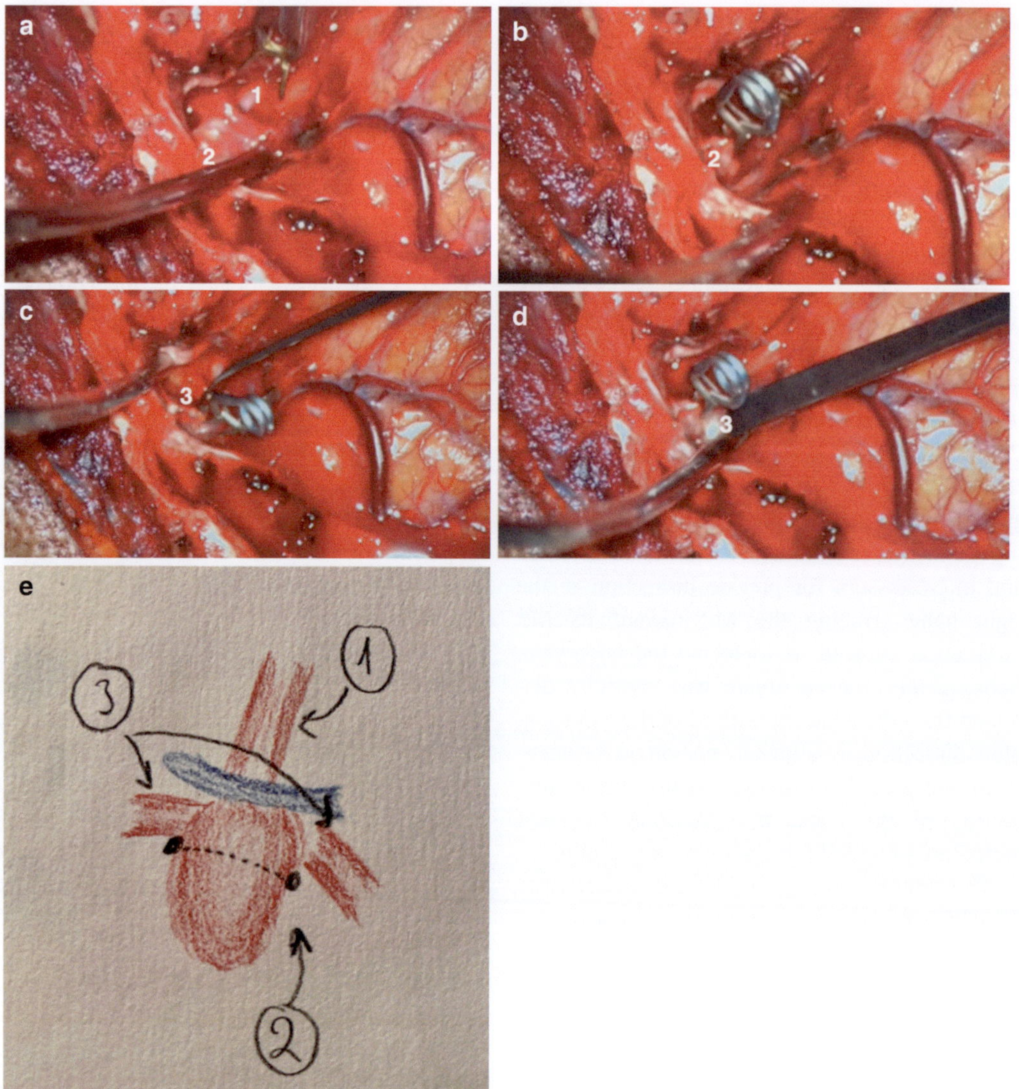

Fig. 7.3 Intraoperative images of microsurgical clipping of the M2-M3 bifurcation aneurysm. The aneurysm was originating from the superior M2 artery trunk. We followed the M2 from the M1-M2 bifurcation all the way distal to the aneurysm. The aneurysm was identified and dissected free in order to define the neck and the arteries coming out of the bifurcation. (**a**) Since the aneurysm is adhered to the brain tissues, a dissection around the aneurysm was safer by temporary occluding the artery of origin (M2) close to the aneurysm neck. (**b**) After temporary clipping of the M2 (2 min temporary clipping time), the neck is dissected aggressively, and since the tension in the aneurysm decreased, a 7 mm slightly curved clip was used to occlude the aneurysm. (**c**) The temporary clip is removed, and the M3 vessels distal to the aneurysm were inspected. The first M3 trunk was inspected for any stenoses caused by the clip. The artery does not seem to be stenosed, and the clip is not too close to the artery. (**d**) The same applies for the other M3 trunk. (**e**) Schematic drawing showing the steps of the clipping procedure. (1) M2 trunk from which the aneurysm originates. The first step was to temporarily occlude this vessel. (2) Aneurysm— aneurysm dissection after temporary occlusion of M2 and the level on which the clip was applied. Attention was paid not to go to close with the clip to the M3s. (3) Both M3 branches. As a third and last step, the M3 branches are inspected to exclude any stenosis of the branches by the clip

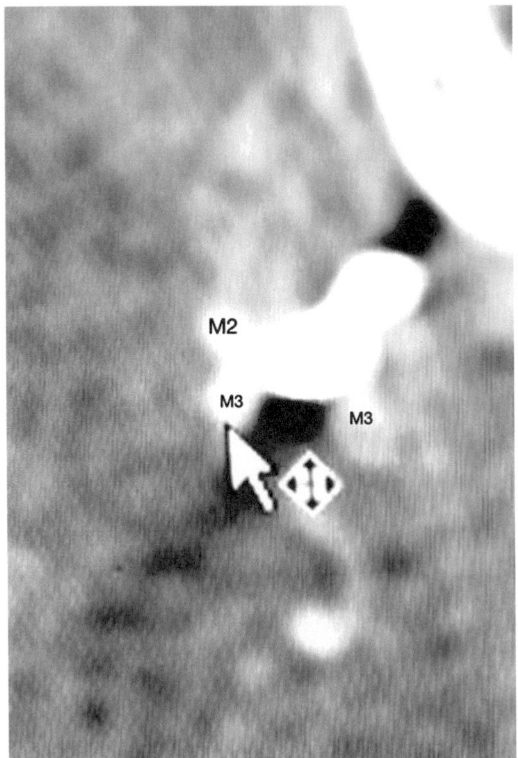

Fig. 7.4 Postoperative CTA of the clipped aneurysm. In this magnified image, the M2 and both M3s can be seen. No infarction is seen in the native cranial CT (image not shown). The aneurysm is not visible indicating a satisfying clip occlusion

The subsequent step involved performing a pterional craniotomy to access and identify the M4 trunk of the frontal lobe. A 1-cm segment was meticulously dissected free, as depicted in Fig. 7.6. An end-to-side STA-M4 anastomosis was executed using 10-0 nonabsorbable sutures. Due to the unavailability of ICG (indocyanine green) or micro-Doppler, we relied on direct observation. The STA exhibited pulsations, while the M4 branch appeared open and uncollapsed (Fig. 7.7).

Following this, we proceeded to open the Sylvian fissure and approached the MCA bifurcation. Notably, the aneurysm was encompassed by scar tissue, necessitating a delicate dissection to free it. Identifying the M1 segment was crucial for achieving proximal control.

Following the liberation of the aneurysm neck, a straight 7-mm clip was employed to occlude it. Dissection around the aneurysm was conducted meticulously, maintaining careful tension on the aneurysm surface to sever it from any adherent arachnoid tissue. However, upon subsequent inspection of the M2 branches, it appeared that the initial clip was causing stenosis in the inferior trunk of the M2. Consequently, we placed an additional slightly curved clip over the first one

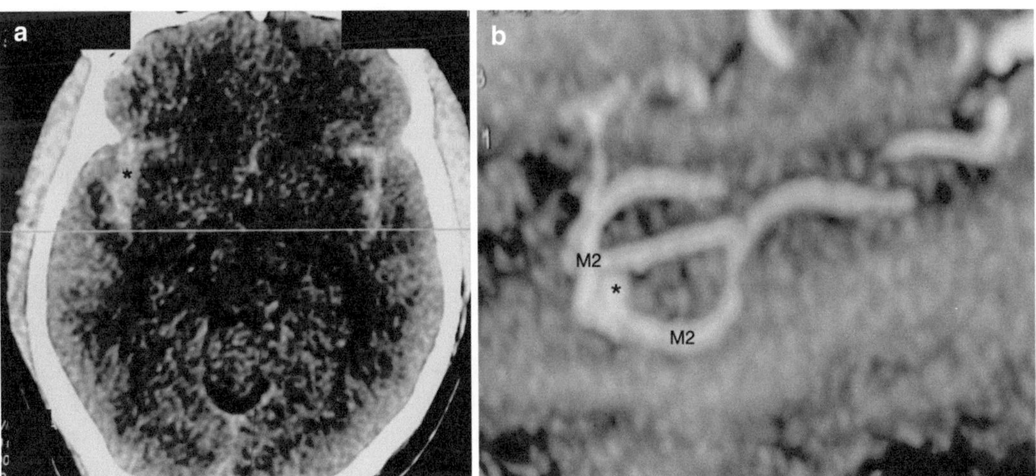

Fig. 7.5 M1-M2 bifurcation aneurysm. A 43-year-old male with ruptured MCA bifurcation aneurysm. The subarachnoid bleeding caused by the aneurysm was 2 months ago. (**a**) Initial native cranial CT shows the SAH with blood in the Sylvian fissures. On the right Sylvian fissure, there was more blood accumulated. (**b**) The CTA shows the MCA bifurcation aneurysm with a probability that the aneurysm originated from the M2 superior trunk (asterisk: aneurysm)

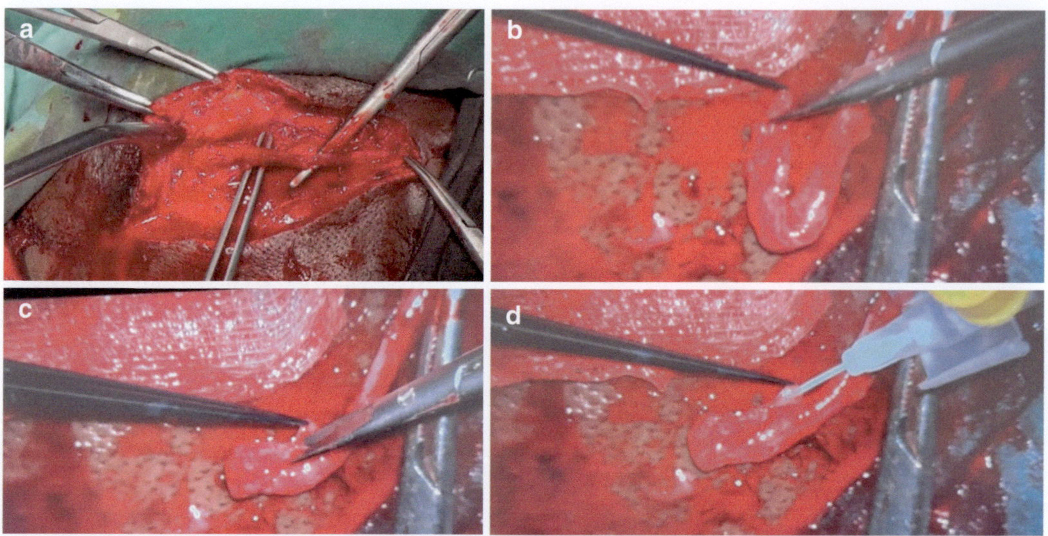

Fig. 7.6 Gathering the donor STA artery for EC-IC bypass. Before clipping of the M1-M2 aneurysm (see Fig. 7.5) was performed, an EC-IC bypass was planned to be placed in case the superior M2 trunk would be occluded during clipping. (**a**) Identification of the STA (parietal branch) from the ear to about 8 cm distally by palpation. Skin cut over the artery and dissection of STA. (**b–d**) Removing perivascular fat, fish-mouthing the artery and rinsing with heparin solution. A temporary clip was placed at the base of the STA close to the ear

and subsequently removed the initial clip to allow space for the M2. This adjustment ensured that the M2 was now free from any stenosis.

The clipping procedure concluded successfully without necessitating sacrifice of the artery from which the aneurysm originated (refer to Fig. 7.8). Figure 7.8 also demonstrates the presence of thick arachnoid tissue observed while opening the Sylvian fissure. Following transportation to the ICU, the patient immediately regained consciousness without experiencing any neurological symptoms.

A postsurgical CTA conducted 1 day postoperation revealed no remaining aneurysms, with reconstructions indicating the integrity of the bypass (see Fig. 7.9). Despite resource limitations, the feasibility of bypass surgery remains viable when required.

Twenty-four hours after the surgery, the patient was transferred to the general ward and was discharged home on the seventh day postoperation.

7.1.3 MCA M2 Fusiform Aneurysm in a Patient with AIDS

There's a prevalent notion among vascular neurosurgeons that performing surgeries on aneurysms in HIV or AIDS patients poses increased difficulty due to the heightened fragility of both the arterial and aneurysmal walls. This impression is shared by our team as well. Despite exercising the utmost caution during dissection around the aneurysm, it has been observed that aneurysms in HIV-positive patients tend to rupture more easily even with minimal manipulation.

In the present case, a female patient diagnosed with a fusiform aneurysm situated on the left M2 segment of the superior trunk. The aneurysm had ruptured 2 days prior to the surgery, resulting in a subarachnoid hemorrhage (SAH) of WFNS grade 2 (refer to Fig. 7.10). It's noteworthy that the inferior trunk was in close proximity to the aneurysm. The primary objective of the surgery was to reconstruct the aneurysm.

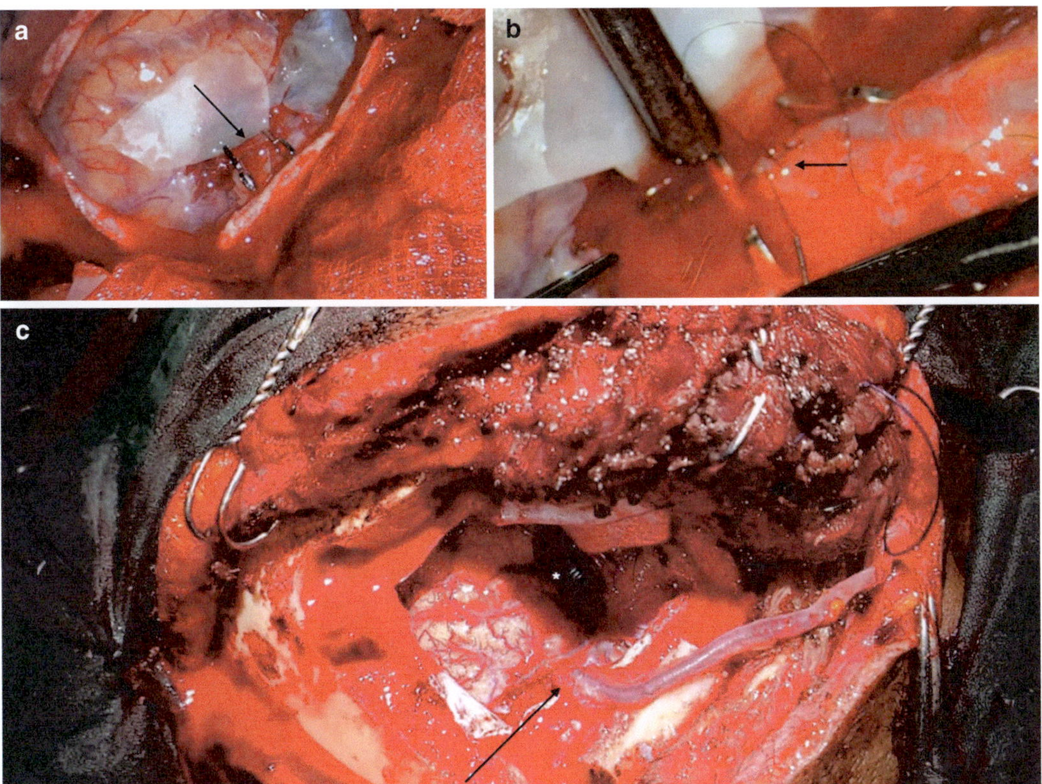

Fig. 7.7 EC-IC bypass before aneurysm clipping. After gathering the STA (see Fig. 7.6), a pterional craniotomy was performed, and an M4 artery of the frontal lobe was identified. (**a**) Dissection of about 1 cm of the M4 artery (arrow). The segment where the arteriotomy will be placed is isolated by two temporary miniclips. (**b**) Suturing the STA artery in an end-to-side fashion to the M4 artery with 10-0 non-resorbable stitches (arrow). (**c**) After the anastomosis is complete first temporary clips from the distal part of the M4 anastomosed artery, the proximal part and then the STA were removed. The STA was filled immediately and pulsated, indicating that the anastomosis was intact (arrow shows the anastomosis location). The picture is taken at the end of surgery where the aneurysm is clipped already (white asterisk indicates the aneurysm clip), and the anastomosis was still intact indicating that no thrombus was built to occlude the STA

A pterional craniotomy was conducted, and the initial dissection around the aneurysm proceeded without any significant incidents. However, while temporarily clipping the M2 proximal to the aneurysm and continuing with further aneurysm dissection, the adjacent inferior trunk of the M2 ruptured at a minimum of two distinct locations.

The extracted aneurysm resulted in two distinct ends of the M2 superior trunk, which unfortunately could not be brought together for an end-to-end anastomosis. Our initial preoperative plan aimed to reconstruct the aneurysm; however, this endeavor failed. As an alternative strategy, if reconstruction failed, the plan was to conduct an end-to-side anastomosis of the M2 superior trunk (as the recipient) to the M2 inferior trunk (as the donor artery). Both strategies faced insurmountable obstacles during the surgical procedure as we encountered unexpectedly high vessel fragility. The vessels tore and bled significantly even with minimal manipulation, rendering both plans unfeasible.

Unexpectedly, we were compelled to occlude the superior trunk of the M2 and cautiously coagulate the torn areas of the inferior trunk of the M2. Fortunately, we observed significant back bleeding from the occluded M2 branch, providing some relief. The patient was awakened in the ICU after 1 day, following the standard practice in Tanzania, since this case was operated in

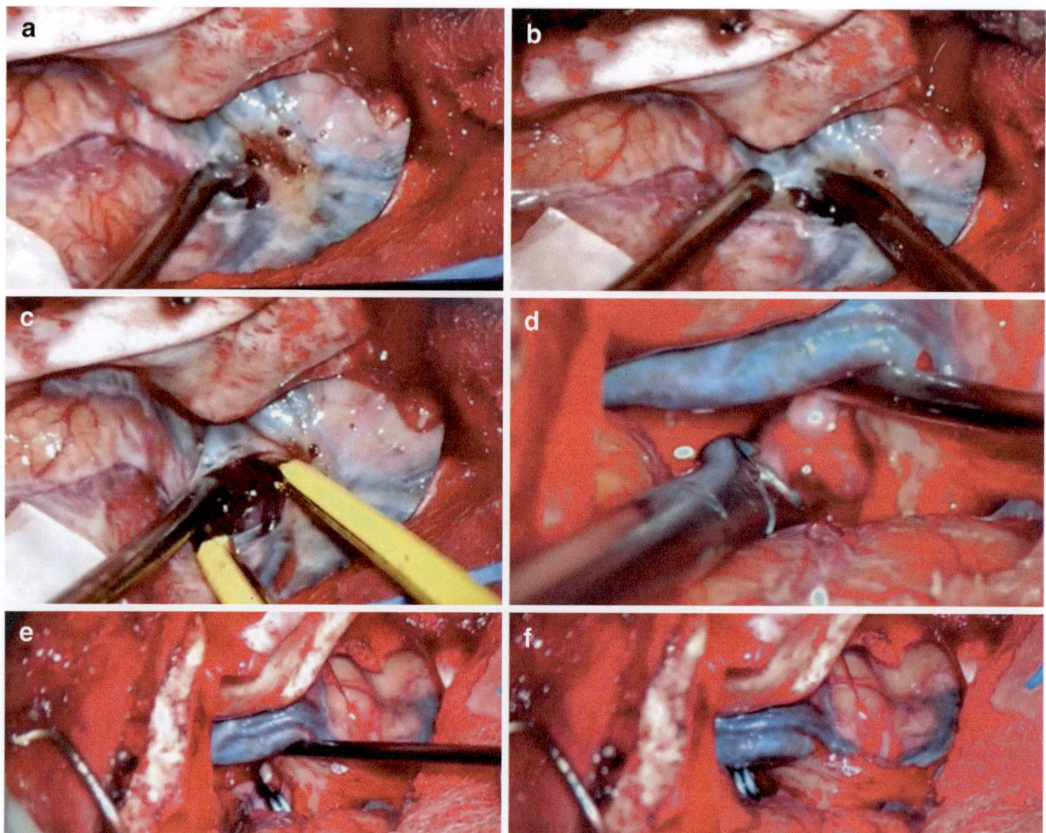

Fig. 7.8 Clipping of the aneurysm after placing an EC-IC bypass. After the bypass (see Fig. 7.7), we proceeded with the M1-M2 aneurysm clipping. (**a**) The Sylvian fissure was opened, but the arachnoid was extreme thick. The aneurysm was ruptured 2 months ago (see Fig. 7.5). Too much blunt dissection and manipulation over the Sylvian fissure could cause a premature re-rupture with catastrophic consequences. Having to deal with arachnoid scar tissue like this forces the surgeon to turn the dissection into a sharp dissection (almost exclusively). Since the patients we are dealing with in Africa had a bleeding some months ago, we have situations with thick arachnoid scar in many cases and in many aneurysms locations (ICA, AcomA, etc.). (**b**) Sharp opening of the Sylvian fissure and careful dissection toward the aneurysm with identification of M3 and M2 arteries. (**c**) After creating a corridor in the arachnoid, the Sylvian fissure is spread with the bipolar forceps. (**d**) The aneurysm is dissected free, the neck is identified, and a 7 mm straight clip is placed to occlude the aneurysm. Even in situations with scar tissue in the arachnoid of the Sylvian fissure, we prefer to approach the aneurysm from distal to proximal (M2-aneurysm-M1) and not from the ICA-M1-M1/M2 bifurcation, which is more traumatic for an already traumatized brain. In a proximal to distal approach, the possibility to use retractors with possible contusions around them is higher. As can be seen in the pictures, we preserve the veins and do not use retractors. (**e**) The clip is 7 mm long which is not the one we would use in the western world. A shorter one would be placed normally, but the available clip armamentarium is limited. We prefer to clip smaller aneurysms with longer clips instead of having clips which are too short to do the job. Since the number of clips we can afford to order is limited, the choice of clips to order has to be taken wisely. (**f**) The clip is placed. Control of aneurysm remnants or stenosis of M2 arteries around the clip is done. End result of the clipping. The Sylvian fissure was opened at a length of about 1.5 cm in order to manipulate and traumatize the brain tissue at minimum. The EC-IC anastomosis (see Fig. 7.7) is under the cottonoid on the right side of the picture

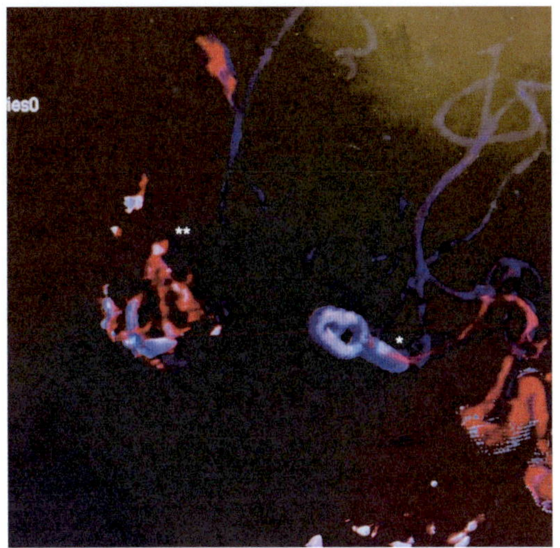

Fig. 7.9 The CTA reconstruction shows no aneurysm (white asterisk) and perfused vessels in the frontal lobe where the anastomosis was placed (double asterisk). More details could not be gained by the reconstruction. The native cranial CT (not shown) shows no infractions, and clinically, the patient had no deficits

Muhimbili University Hospital, dar es Salaam. However, the current objective is to extubate patients immediately postsurgery to enable immediate clinical assessment. Postsurgery, the patient presented with right-hand paralysis, and the subsequent postoperative CTA revealed no perfusion of the M2s (Fig. 7.11).

Ten days after the surgery, she suffered from pneumocystis carinii pneumonia and passed away. Planning bypass procedures in patients with HIV angiopathy can easily lead to a disaster. If the patient doesn't have subarachnoid hemorrhage (SAH), we would be highly skeptical about electively clipping and anastomosing fusiform aneurysms in HIV patients where angiopathy is suspected. Given this complex situation with various sometimes unpredictable variables, microsurgical treatment of fusiform aneurysms in HIV-positive patients, especially in cases of AIDS, should be carefully reconsidered on an individual basis.

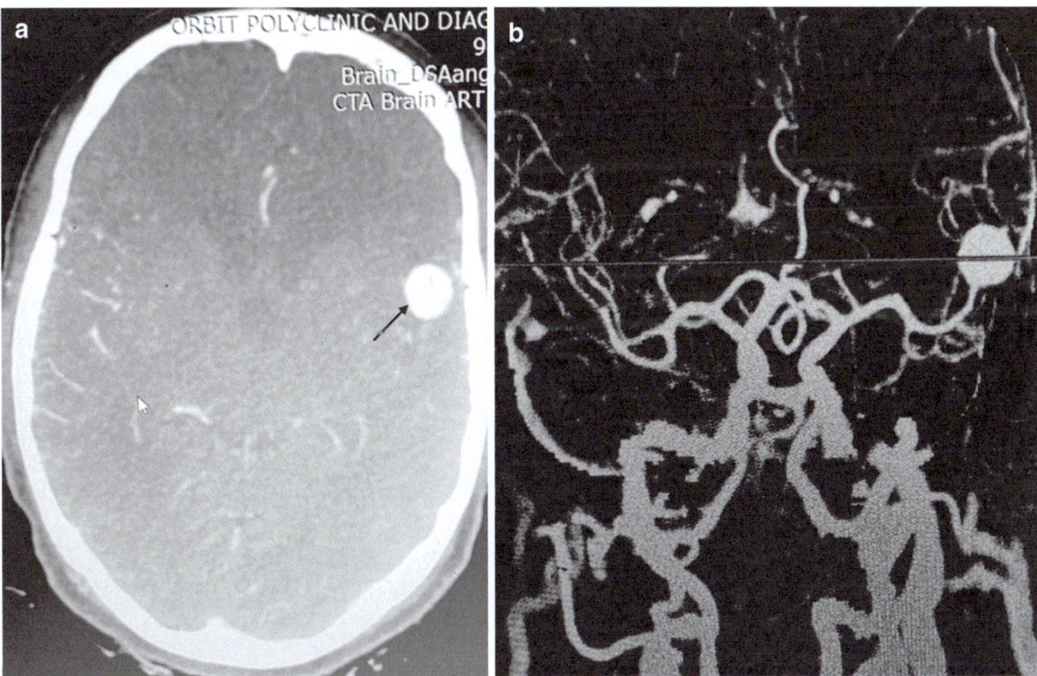

Fig. 7.10 Ruptured M2 fusiform aneurysm in a patient with AIDS. The patient suffered an SAH 2 days ago (WFNS 3). (**a**) CTA shows an aneurysm (arrow) of the M2 artery as the reason of the SAH. (**b**) The CTA reconstruction indicates a fusiform aneurysm. At least one branch of the M2 leaves the aneurysm on its distal end. The M2 goes into the aneurysm at a 7 o'clock position, and there is another part of the M2 vessel leaving the aneurysm at a 1 o'clock position

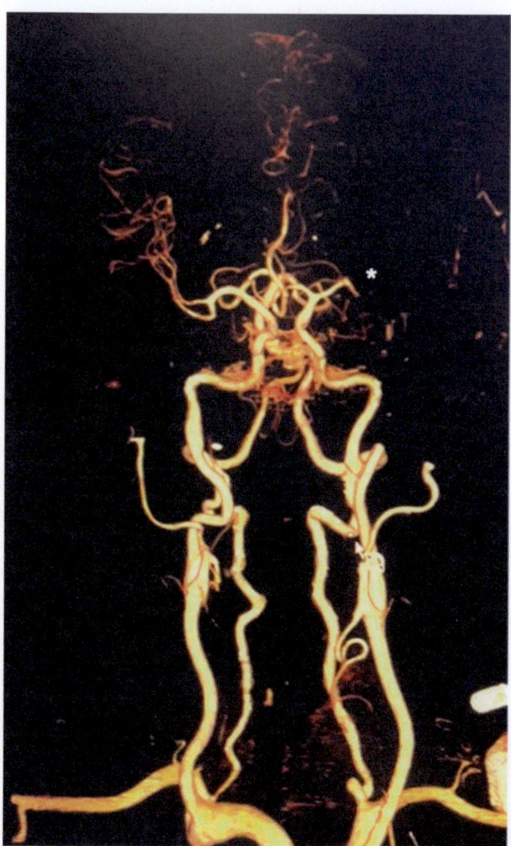

Fig. 7.11 Postoperative CTA of the clipped MCA aneurysm of Fig. 7.10. This coronal CTA reconstruction shows a perfusion stop of the left MCA artery. The asterisk indicates the position of the clip. These patient suffered an MCA infarction with plegia of her right hand

7.2   Clipping of Internal Carotid Artery (ICA) Aneurysms

7.2.1   Complex Posterior Wall ICA Aneurysm

A 45-year-old female patient was scheduled for surgery due to a non-bleeding aneurysm with no neurological deficits, except for visual weakness in her right eye. Preoperative cerebral CTA revealed an aneurysm, likely originating from the right internal carotid artery (ICA) and exerting pressure on the posterior aspect of the right A1.

In the CTA images, there was uncertainty regarding whether the aneurysm originated from the A1 or the ICA (refer to Fig. 7.12). Consequently, the artery where the aneurysm neck originated needed intraoperative exploration, since DSA was unavailable.

The patient's head was secured in a head holder (rotated 40° to the left, retroflexed 20°, and inclined 20° anti-Trendelenburg). We accessed the aneurysm using a subfrontal-pterional approach. Before opening the dura, an external ventricular drainage was inserted into the right ventricle. Upon opening the dura mater, we observed brain swelling, prompting us to alleviate the pressure by draining approximately 30 mL of cerebrospinal fluid (CSF) from the lateral ventricle.

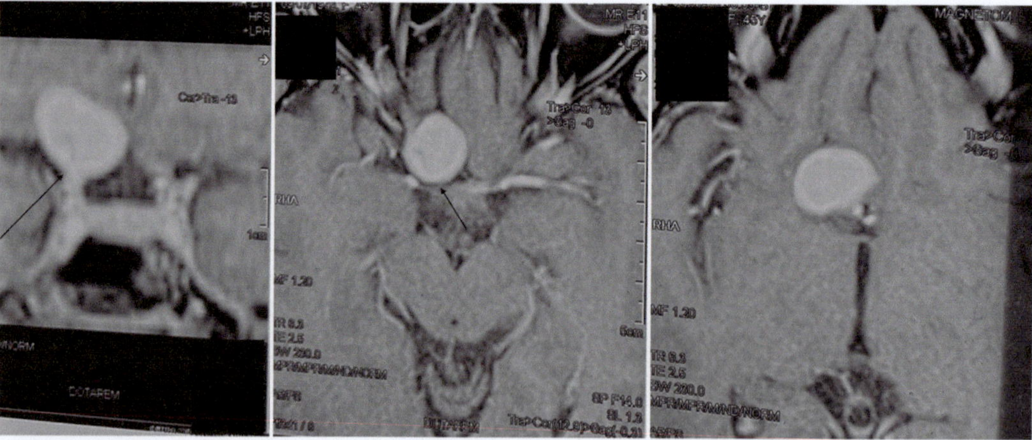

Fig. 7.12 Complex ICA aneurysm in a 45-year-old female. Coronal and transverse MRA sections of the giant aneurysm (arrow). The aneurysm was not ruptured. The coronal section indicates the aneurysm to originate from the ICA. Some doubt is risen though since the artery of aneurysm origin could be the A1. Having these images for diagnosis and without DSA, the dissection of the aneurysm and the ICA and A1 has to be very careful in order to not penetrate the aneurysm neck by accident

We drained an adequate amount of cerebrospinal fluid (CSF) until reaching a point where approaching the carotid cistern became feasible without difficulty. The use of retractors is significantly limited in our procedures. In rare instances involving anterior communicating artery (AcomA) aneurysms, retractors are utilized briefly, usually for a few minutes, primarily to position the clip. Our primary objective during the fellowship training is to equip fellows with the skills to perform surgeries without relying on retractors. The technique involves retracting the brain using suction in the left hand while manipulating a dissector or other instruments with the right hand.

Given the substantial size of the aneurysm, our initial dissection targeted the area around it.

Initially, we identified the A1, presuming it to be the point of origin for the aneurysm. However, upon dissecting the aneurysm from the A1, no visible neck was observed on this vessel. Proceeding from distal to proximal, we dissected the internal carotid artery (ICA), and in close proximity to the ophthalmic artery, we successfully identified the aneurysm neck. Subsequently, the aneurysm was occluded using a straight 9 mm clip.

There was no residual perfusion observed in the aneurysm (refer to Fig. 7.13). The cranial bone was repositioned and secured solely with stitches in an X-shaped pattern. Following surgery, the patient spent 1 night in the ICU and then 4 days in the peripheral ward. Subsequent postoperative CTA scans displayed no filling of the

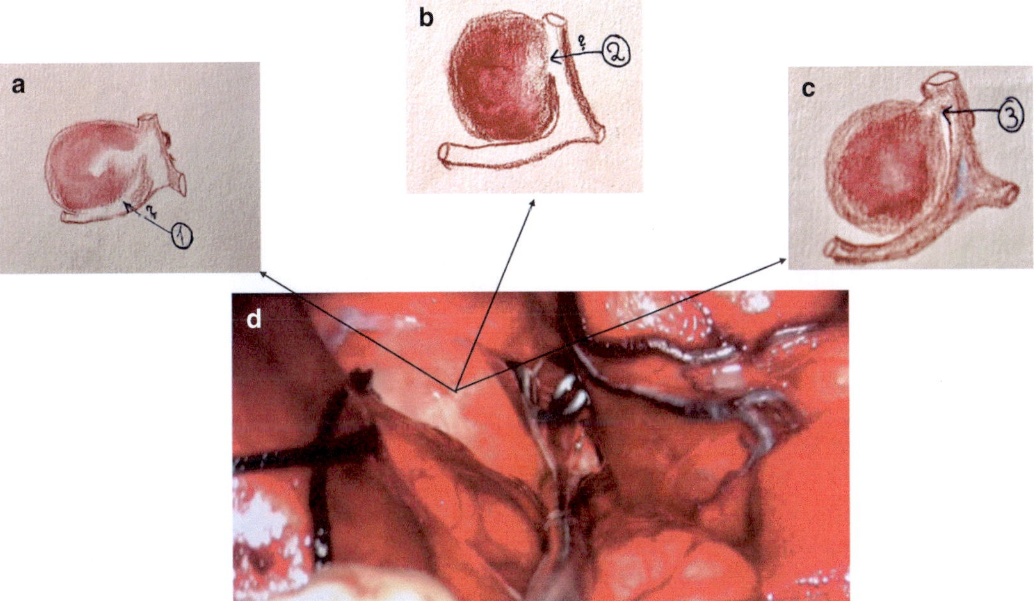

Fig. 7.13 Presurgical drawing planning the surgical steps. In complex cases, we recommend to draw a surgical plan which should be followed. This allows the surgeon to mentally draw a picture of the anticipating anatomy and have a clear plan. The drawing takes some time to think and to focus into details. (**a**) At first it was planned to dissect the A1 (1) in order to find out if the aneurysm originated from this artery. (**b**) Should the aneurysm not originate from the A1, the ICA would be dissected free from the ophthalmic artery to the ICA bifurcation (2) in order to identify the aneurysm neck. (**c**) The aneurysm neck was identified between the ophthalmic artery and the pcoma. The neck of the aneurysm was narrow (3). (**d**) The aneurysm could be easily occluded with one straight 9 mm clip

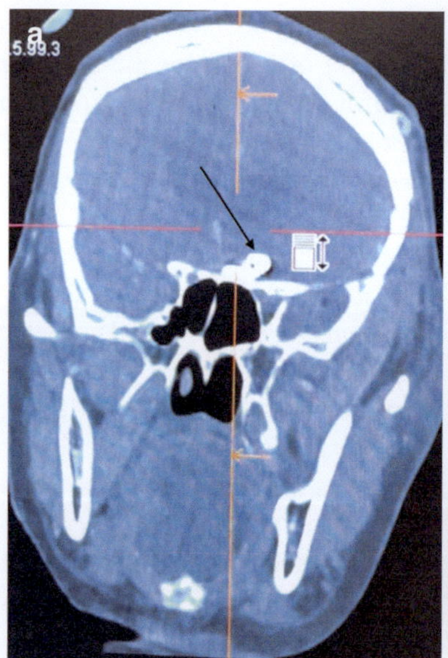
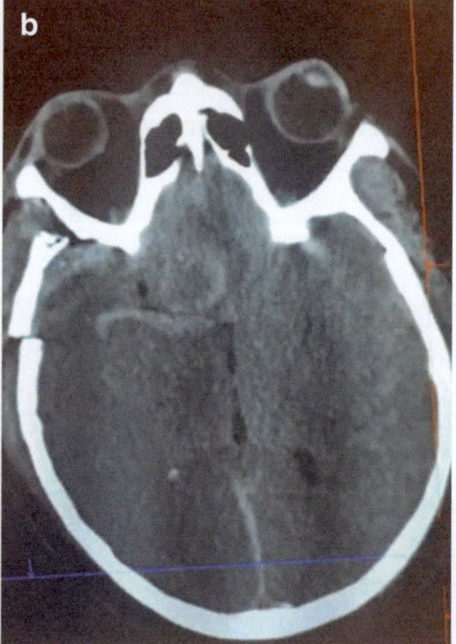

Fig. 7.14 An unpredictable catastrophic event. (**a**) The postsurgical course of the patient was uneventful. She was extubated immediately after surgery and had no neurologic deficits. As shown in the coronal reconstruction of her CTA, the aneurysm was occluded (arrow indicates the clip). She was discharged from the hospital at day 5. (**b**) When at home (ninth postoperative day), the patient fell in her bathroom. In the CCT immediately after the fall, subarachnoid blood and brain edema can be seen, which pushes the craniotomy bone outward. Unfortunately, the patient died as a consequence of her fall

aneurysm post clip occlusion. The carotid perfusion was satisfactory, and no signs of infarction were evident (Fig. 7.14).

However, after returning home, she likely experienced a seizure and fell in the bathroom, sustaining head injuries on the craniotomy side. It appeared that during the fall, the bone became embedded in the brain tissue. A CT scan performed by a peripheral hospital showed blood in the subarachnoid spaces (Fig. 7.14). The patient was intubated by colleagues and transferred to the reference hospital where the clipping was initially performed. There were issues with the intubation tube placement in the esophagus, requiring re-intubation. Subsequently, the patient lost consciousness and unfortunately passed away a few hours after admission.

This case marks the only postoperative mortality within 10 days in our series which was

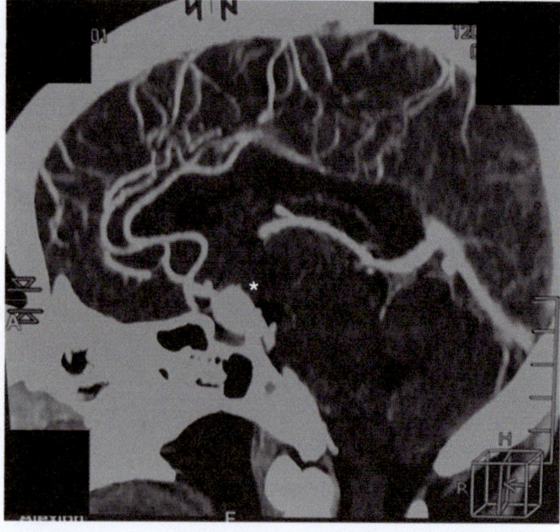

Fig. 7.15 Fusiform ruptured ICA aneurysm in a 56-year-old female patient. The sagittal CTA reconstruction shows the fusiform ICA aneurysm (asterisk). It was planned to clip-reconstruct the aneurysm, which can be seen in Fig. 7.16

caused by direct surgical complications. It's important to note that there were no intraoperative mortalities. The surgeries incurred moderate blood loss, eliminating the need for blood transfusion from the blood bank.

7.2.2 Clip Reconstructed Fusiform ICA Aneurysm

A 56-year-old female patient, who had a WFNS 1 SAH 6 weeks prior, was admitted for clip occlusion of a fusiform aneurysm located in the left internal carotid artery (Fig. 7.15). Unfortunately, at that time, the microinstruments necessary for bypass surgery were unavailable. Consequently, the sole treatment option was clip reconstruction. If this approach failed, the alternative considered was carotid occlusion. The hope was that the contralateral side would provide adequate flow to perfuse the affected hemisphere.

The patient's head was secured in the head holder with a 30° leftward tilt and a 35° retroflexion. Additionally, the body was inclined at a 20° anti-Trendelenburg angle. To induce brain relaxation, 20% Mannitol (150 mL) was administered, and systolic blood pressure was maintained below 110 mmHg. Before opening the dura, an external ventricular drain (EVD) was inserted to ensure sufficient relaxation, facilitating retractorless dissection along the skull base toward the optic nerve and the internal carotid artery (ICA) Following dissection of the anterior aspect of the ICA, both the posterior communicating artery (PCOM) and the choroidal artery were identified, revealing the aneurysm situated on the posterior wall of the ICA.

For the clip reconstruction, a 90° fenestrated ring clip was utilized (Fig. 7.16). This particular fenestrated clip serves as a fundamental component in our aneurysm clip arsenal, particularly applied for aneurysms situated on posterior artery walls. As a precautionary measure, the internal carotid artery (ICA) was temporarily clipped proximal to the aneurysm. The clipping procedure was successful. Unfortunately, due to financial constraints, the patient's family couldn't afford a postoperative CTA to verify the surgical outcome.

This is just one example of the financial burden placed on affected individuals. This family gathered all their funds to afford a potentially life-saving operation for their beloved mother. Due to financial constraints and their trust in the surgical team that the operation would be successful, they were unable to undergo the crucial postoperative follow-up that is essential in our countries.

7.2.3 A. Choroidea ICA Aneurysm on the Left ICA and Posterior Wall Left pcomA Aneurysm

A 64-year-old female patient who experienced SAH WFNS grade 1 3 weeks ago was admitted for aneurysm clip occlusion. The CTA was conducted at another hospital, and the image quality was suboptimal with thick slices (Fig. 7.17). Nevertheless, a left ICA aneurysm was apparent, located on its posterior wall. For the clip occlusion, our plan involved using fenestrated clips to facilitate the placement of the ICA into the fenestration. Patient positioning and brain relaxation were achieved as described in Sect. 7.2.2.

A subfrontal approach was selected. As the dissection of the ICA proceeded from the ophthalmic artery to the ICA bifurcation, a second aneurysm involving the anterior choroidal artery became apparent, which had not been detected in the MRA. This aneurysm was clipped using an angled clip, as depicted in Fig. 7.18. This approach was deemed optimal to facilitate the clipping of the larger ICA aneurysm without interference from the clip used on the anterior choroidal artery aneurysm. The goal was to prevent the clip on the anterior choroidal artery aneurysm from impeding the placement of the

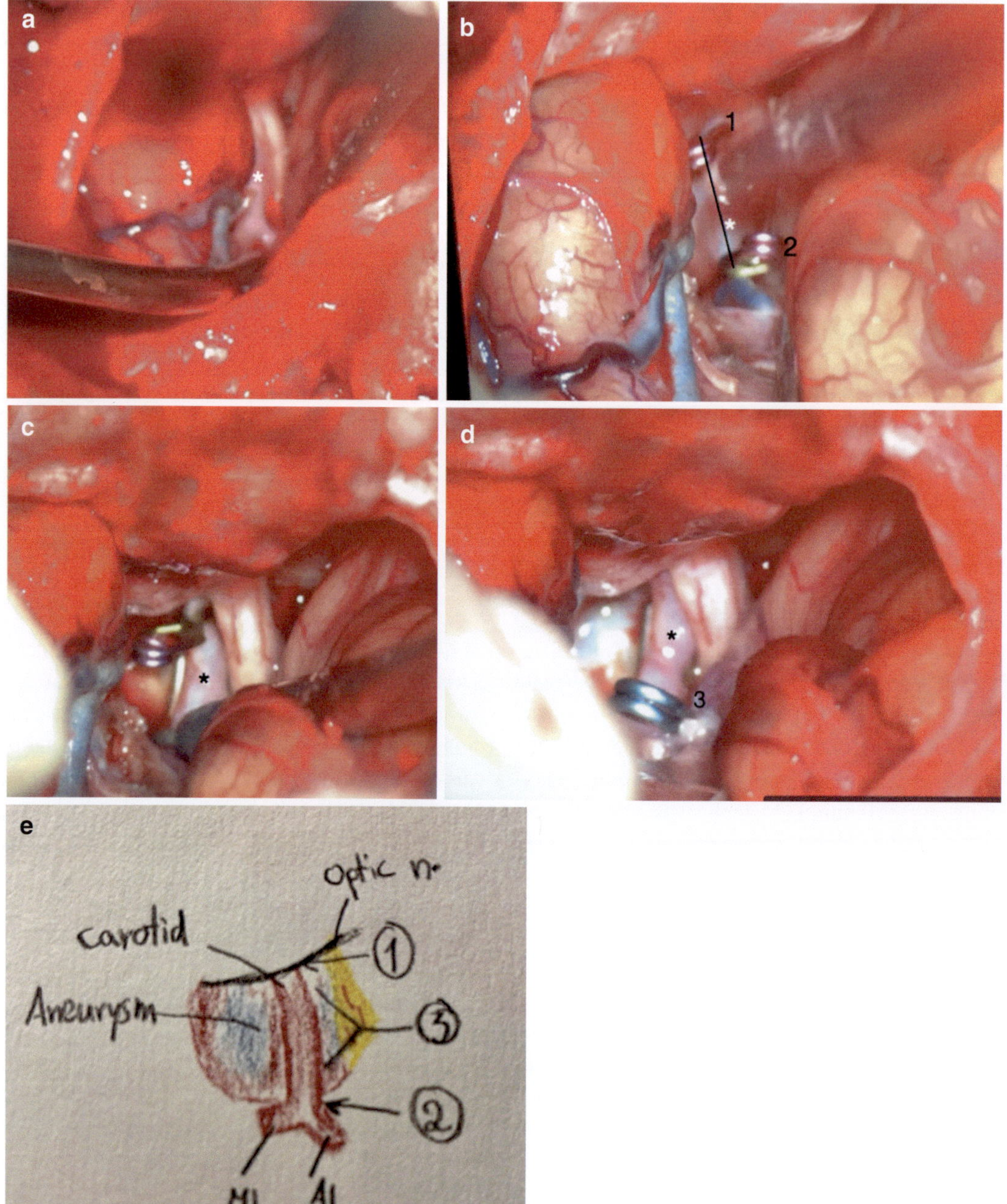

Fig. 7.16 Clipping of the broad necked ICA aneurysm of Fig. 7.15. (**a**) Subfrontal dissection to the ICA (asterisk) from the ophthalmic artery origin to the ICA bifurcation. (**b**) After dissecting the ICA in its intradural segment, temporary clips were placed close to the ophthalmic artery origin (1) and to the ICA bifurcation (2). The black line shows the anticipated length of the aneurysm neck. The aneurysm was not fusiform but broad necked, which made clip occlusion easier. (**c**) After temporary clipping of the ICA which trapped the aneurysm (except the pcoma which was left open, the aneurysm was identified in the posterior wall of the ICA (asterisk). (**d**) The aneurysm neck is dissected in its whole length and could be clip occluded with a 90° angulated fenestrated clip (3). The ICA (asterisk) was passing through the fenestration. (**e**) Schematic drawing of the surgical image. (1) The position of the first temporary clip, (2) the position of the second temporary clip, (3) position of the permanent aneurysm clip

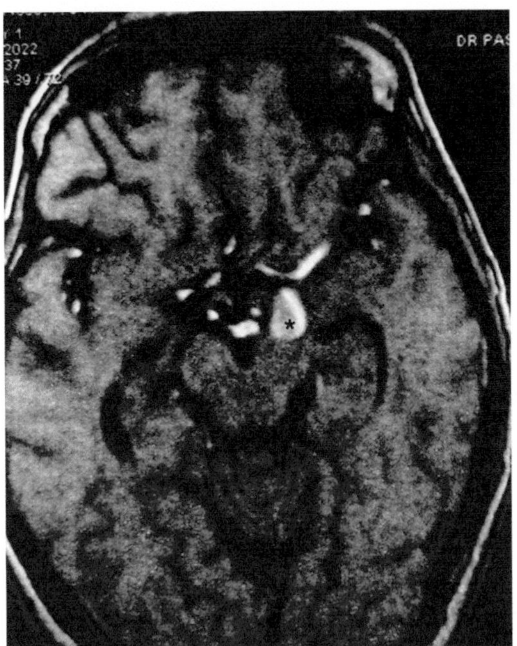

Fig. 7.17 Art. choroidal ICA aneurysms on the left ICA and posterior wall pcomA aneurysm. The MRA shows ICA aneurysm on this 64-year-old female patient, which ruptured 3 weeks before surgery. This image was the only one showing the aneurysm. The slices where too thick, and since we saw clearly the aneurysm, we proceeded to the surgical clipping, without further new or additional imaging (asterisk: aneurysm)

clip on the adjacent aneurysm, which was in close proximity to the posterior communicating artery (pcom). Due to the presence of scar tissue surrounding both aneurysms and the challenging dissection of the neck, the definitive clip placement was conducted subsequent to temporary occlusion of the ICA.

Various sizes of temporary clips are essential components of a fundamental clip armamentarium. After successfully clipping the anterior choroidal artery ICA aneurysm, it was meticulously opened and verified to confirm complete occlusion. Subsequently, attention shifted to the aneurysm situated distal to the posterior communicating artery (pcom) and proximal to the anterior choroidal artery, where the neck was clearly identified (Fig. 7.18). To occlude this aneurysm, a 90° fenestrated clip was employed, positioned in accordance with Fig. 7.18. Initially, during the attempt to clip and position the carotid into the fenestration, it appeared that the direction of the clip caused stenosis in the internal carotid artery (ICA). Consequently, the clip's direction was altered to prevent ICA stenosis. However, the neck remained incompletely occluded, and upon further examination, a small remnant was detected distal to the clip. To address this, a straight fenestrated clip was used in addition to the 90° fenestrated clip. During the assessment of the clip's position around the aneurysm, the aneurysm ruptured due to the displacement of the straight clip from the aneurysm neck. Subsequently, temporary occlusion of the ICA was necessary, and the straight clip was repositioned closer to the angulated clip, as depicted in Fig. 7.18. The hemorrhage ceased, and the surgical site was closed. Four hours postsurgery, the patient was extubated in the ICU, but she experienced a contralateral hemiparesis. A follow-up CCT/CTA revealed an infarction in the anterior choroidal artery territory, likely explaining the observed neurological symptoms (Fig. 7.19).

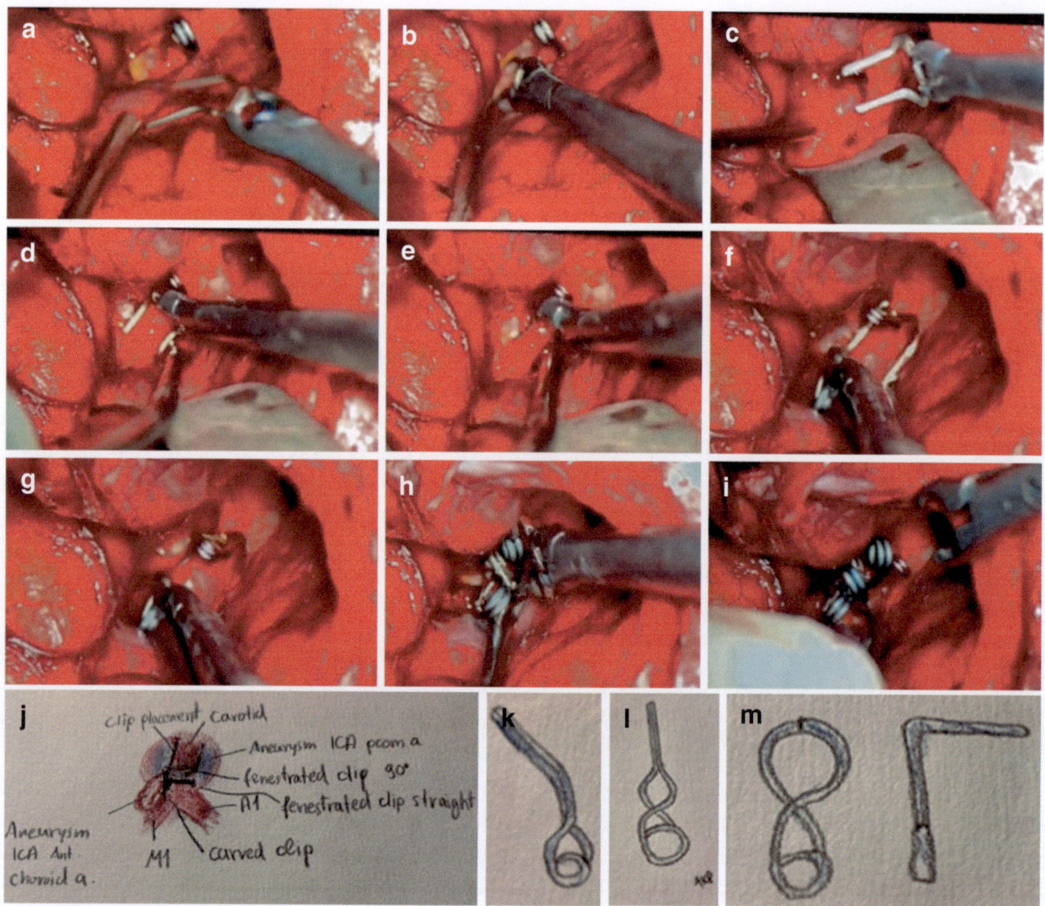

Fig. 7.18 Clipping of two aneurysms in the intradural ICA. A 64-year-old female patient with SAH 3 weeks ago. The MRA showed one ICA aneurysm which was the culprit of the bleeding. After clipping, both aneurysms were opened to assure complete occlusion. (**a** and **b**) Subfrontal approach to the ICA and dissection of the vessel over its complete intradural course. Instead of one aneurysm on the posterior wall of the ICA, a second one could be identified which was originating close to the ant. choroidal artery. This aneurysm had a narrow neck and was clipped with an angulated clip as shown in (**k**). This clip would not interfere with the clipping of the broad necked second ICA aneurysm. The second aneurysm took us by surprise, since it was not seen in the MRA. (**c–e**) For the clipping of the posterior wall aneurysm (see also (**j**)), a fenestrated clip was used at first. Placement of the clip in the direction shown in the picture leads to a stenosis of the ICA (**e**), and therefore the clip was removed again. (**f–i**) Temporary clipping of the proximal ICA close to the ophthalmic artery origin and second attempt of clip occlude the aneurysm with the fenestrated 90° angulated clip in the opposite direction as shown in (**c–e**) in order to place the clip further away from the ICA to prevent ICA stenosis. The clip application was successful, and a small aneurysm remnant could be seen, which caused aneurysm filling. This part of the aneurysm was clipped by a straight fenestrated clip. (**j**) Drawing of the surgical field. (**k**) The angulated clip used to clip-occlude the ICA-ant. choroidal artery aneurysm. (**l**) Fenestrated straight clip which was used to occlude a remnant of the posterior wall ICA aneurysm. (**m**) Fenestrated 90° angulated clip to occlude the main part of the neck of the posterior wall ICA aneurysm

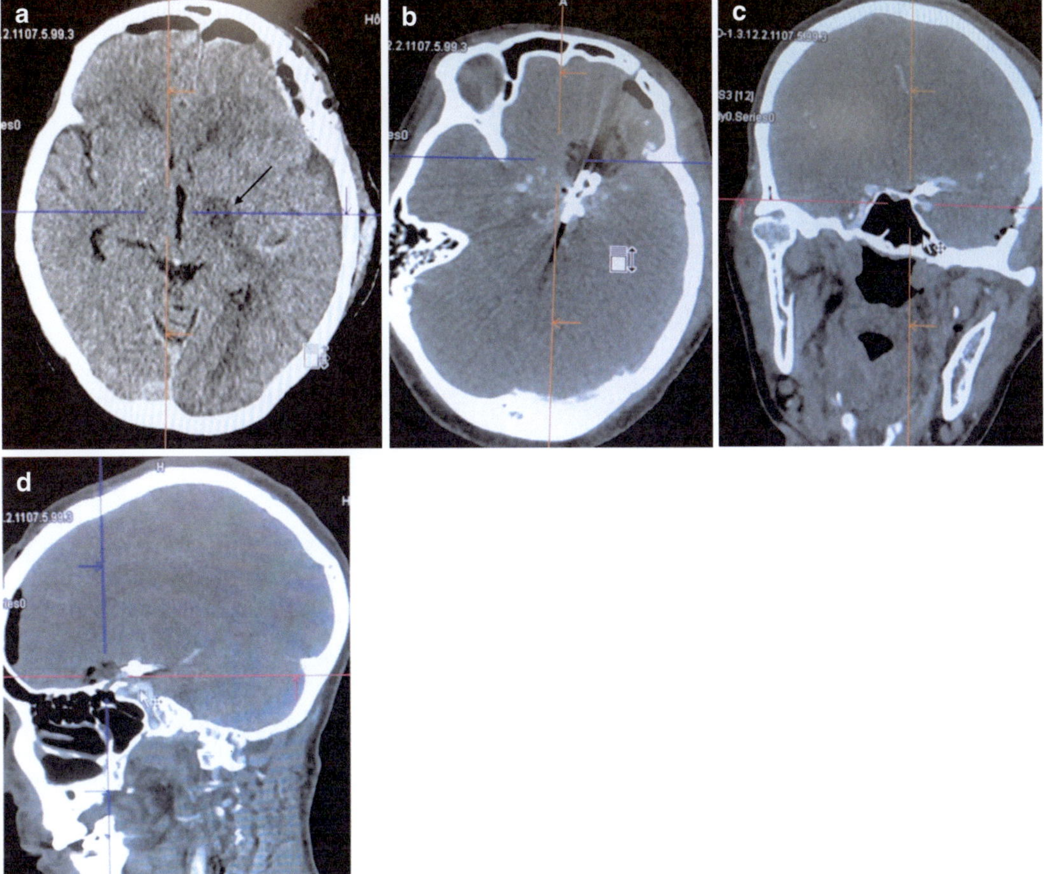

Fig. 7.19 Postoperative CCT and CTA of the patient with 2 ICA aneurysms (see Figs. 7.17 and 7.18). (**a**) The postoperative native cranial CT of the patient shows an infarction of the ant. choroidal artery on the left side (arrow). Clinically the patient suffered a hemipalsy on the right side. Intraoperatively, the choroidal artery was intact, and the clip was not contacting or stenosing the vessel. However, the temporary clipping of the ICA lasted 25 min, which could also be a reason of the choroidal infarction (combined with the clip application close to the vessel). ICG control intraoperatively would help to recognize this problem and maybe prevent the high morbidity we caused during this surgery. Only visual control of the vessels and placing the clip as far away as possible off the arteries and still having a satisfying occlusion of the aneurysms can fail in small caliber vessels like the ant. choroidal art. with a high price for patient and doctor. (**b–d**) Transverse (**b**), coronal (**c**), and sagittal (**d**) sections of the postoperative CTA showing no aneurysms (complete occlusion)

7.3 Clip Occlusion of Anterior Communicating Artery (AcomA) Aneurysms

7.3.1 Left Side A1-A2 Aneurysm and a Right-Sided Proximal A2 Aneurysm in a HIV-Positive Patient

A 42-year-old female patient presented with a subarachnoid hemorrhage (SAH) classified as WFNS grade 2, experienced 14 days prior. Her HIV-positive status suggested a certain level of vasculopathy. A detailed reconstruction from the CTA indicated the presence of an A1-A2 aneurysm on the left side and a proximal A2 artery aneurysm on the right side (see Fig. 7.20). Determining which aneurysm was the source of the bleeding solely from the CTA proved challenging. However, this ambiguity did not alter our approach. In cases involving multiple aneurysms with limited diagnostic imaging such as CTA, each aneurysm is managed as potentially contributing to the bleeding. The patient's posi-

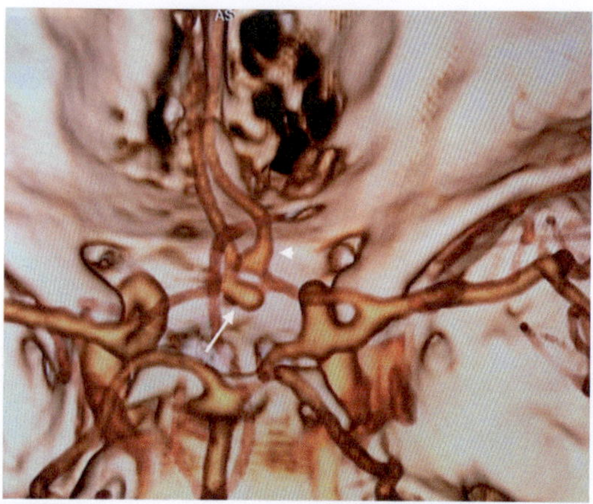

Fig. 7.20 HIV positive patient with an A1-A2 aneurysm left and a proximal A2 aneurysm right. The 42-year-old female patient suffered an SAH 2 weeks ago. The CTA revealed 2 aneurysms and no vasospasms. One aneurysm was located on the left proximal A2 (arrowhead), and the second one was located on the A1-A2 junction (arrow). The approach we planned was subfrontal right

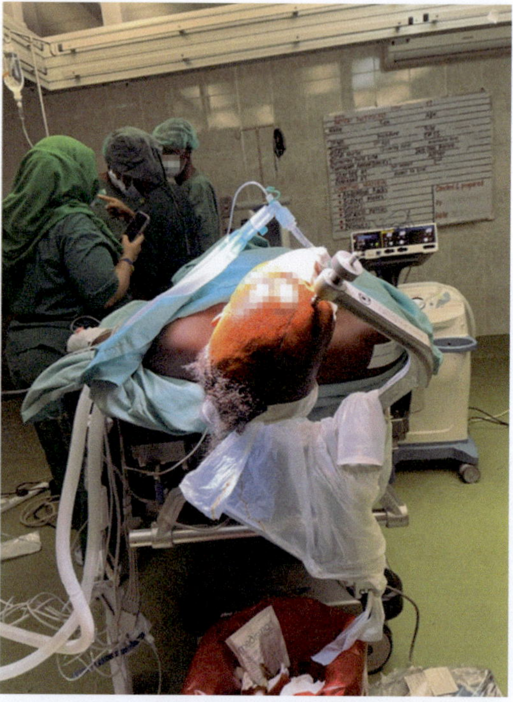

Fig. 7.21 Positioning of the patient for AcomA aneurysm clipping. Head fixation with a retroflexion of about 25°, rotation to the right of 30–40°, and anti-Trendelenburg of 20°. This position allows the brain to move away from the skull base by gravitation and avoid any use of retractors. It is important for the surgeon to know exactly how the head is positioned, since an EVD will be placed during surgery. Even when the positioning is performed by the residents or fellows, the surgeon has to see the position of the head before sterile drapes cover the patient. After that you can drink your coffee for a couple of minutes

tioning during the surgical procedure is depicted in Fig. 7.21.

After the craniotomy, an external ventricular drain (EVD) was inserted into the left lateral ventricle before proceeding to open the dura (see Fig. 7.22). A subfrontal approach was chosen for the procedure. Initially, identification of the optic nerve was followed by a lateral incision to access the carotid cistern. Dissection of the carotid artery was meticulously carried out to gain proximal control, intending to regulate blood flow in case of a potential re-rupture of the aneurysms. The left-side A1 was located over which dissection of the A1s and A2s was conducted.

Both aneurysms were successfully located; yet, consistent with observations in HIV-positive patients, they exhibited a high degree of fragility and ruptured easily during minimal manipulation. To manage the bleeding, cottonoid was gently applied with slight pressure to the ruptured sites, effectively halting the hemorrhage. This allowed for continued dissection around the aneurysms to better understand their anatomy, particularly identifying the location of the neck. Despite these challenges, both aneurysms were successfully clipped without the need for temporary clipping of any of the A1s.

The aneurysms were incised to confirm their complete occlusion, given the unavailability of ICG or micro-Doppler during the surgery (refer to Fig. 7.23 for the surgical illustration). Following the procedure, the patient was successfully extubated in the operating room and demonstrated full movement in all four extremities. Upon admission to the intensive care unit (ICU), there were no apparent neurological deficits, and the postoperative CTA revealed no remaining aneurysms, exhibiting excellent perfusion in both A2 segments. Furthermore, no signs of infarction were observed (Fig. 7.24).

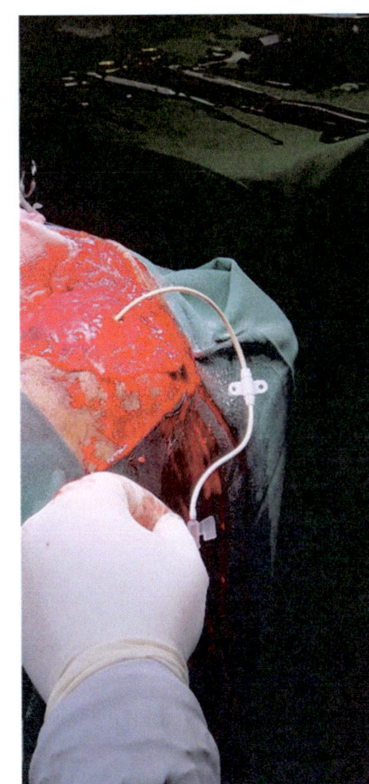

Fig. 7.22 Intraoperatively and after craniotomy, but before opening the dura, we place an external ventricular drainage in the lateral ventricle, which remains closed. After that, the dura is opened in a C-shaped fashion for a subfrontal approach. We check how much pressure has the brain and drain as much CSF as needed in order to approach the optic nerve and the ICA. We prefer the use of EVD instead of lumbar drainage, which is not draining CSF as fast as we need and is unreliable (personal experience, not evidence based). If there are no signs of hydrocephalus before surgery, we remove the EVD in the OR immediately after aneurysm clipping in order to avoid any infections

7.3.2   Complex Left Anterior Communicating Artery (AcomA) Aneurysm Adhering to the Frontopolar and Right A1 Artery

A 56-year-old male patient experienced a WFNS grade 3 SAH resulting from a ruptured AcomA aneurysm, as evident in the CTA scan (see Fig. 7.25). Following appropriate head positioning and brain relaxation facilitated by mannitol administration, systolic blood pressure control,

and an existing EVD, already positioned in the ICU, a pterional craniotomy was conducted.

The surgical procedure is depicted in Fig. 7.26. The Sylvian fissure was opened to create space, and dissection around the optic nerve was performed. Upon opening the carotid cistern, the ipsilateral A1 was identified and dissected toward the aneurysm. Identifying the aneurysm's neck was challenging due to its larger size compared to what was observed in the CTA (about 50% of the aneurysm was thrombosed). The contralateral A1 and the frontopolar artery were adhered to the aneurysm. Dissection was meticulously conducted near the planned clip position to safeguard the frontopolar and A1 vessels. Using a straight 9 mm clip, the aneurysm was occluded, and its interior was inspected to ensure complete occlusion. The thrombotic material within the aneurysm was removed. Following surgery, the patient was extubated in the operating room and subsequently transferred to the ICU. Postoperative CTA demonstrated normal perfusion in all vessels and no signs of perfusion deficits (Fig. 7.27).

7.3.3   Ruptured AcomA Aneurysm with Adhesion to the Arachnoid Tissue

A 48-year-old male patient experienced an SAH resulting from a ruptured AcomA aneurysm 3 months ago (Fig. 7.28). He was admitted for surgery. The approach to the aneurysm was from the right side. The patient's head was secured in the head holder, rotated 20° to the left, and retroflexed 30°, and an EVD was inserted. Mannitol was administered, and systolic blood pressure was maintained below 110 mmHg, following the protocols detailed in previous cases. After opening the dura, we released sufficient CSF to facilitate access to the optic nerve and the carotid without utilizing retractors.

A supraorbital craniotomy was performed, and the carotid cistern was opened to facilitate

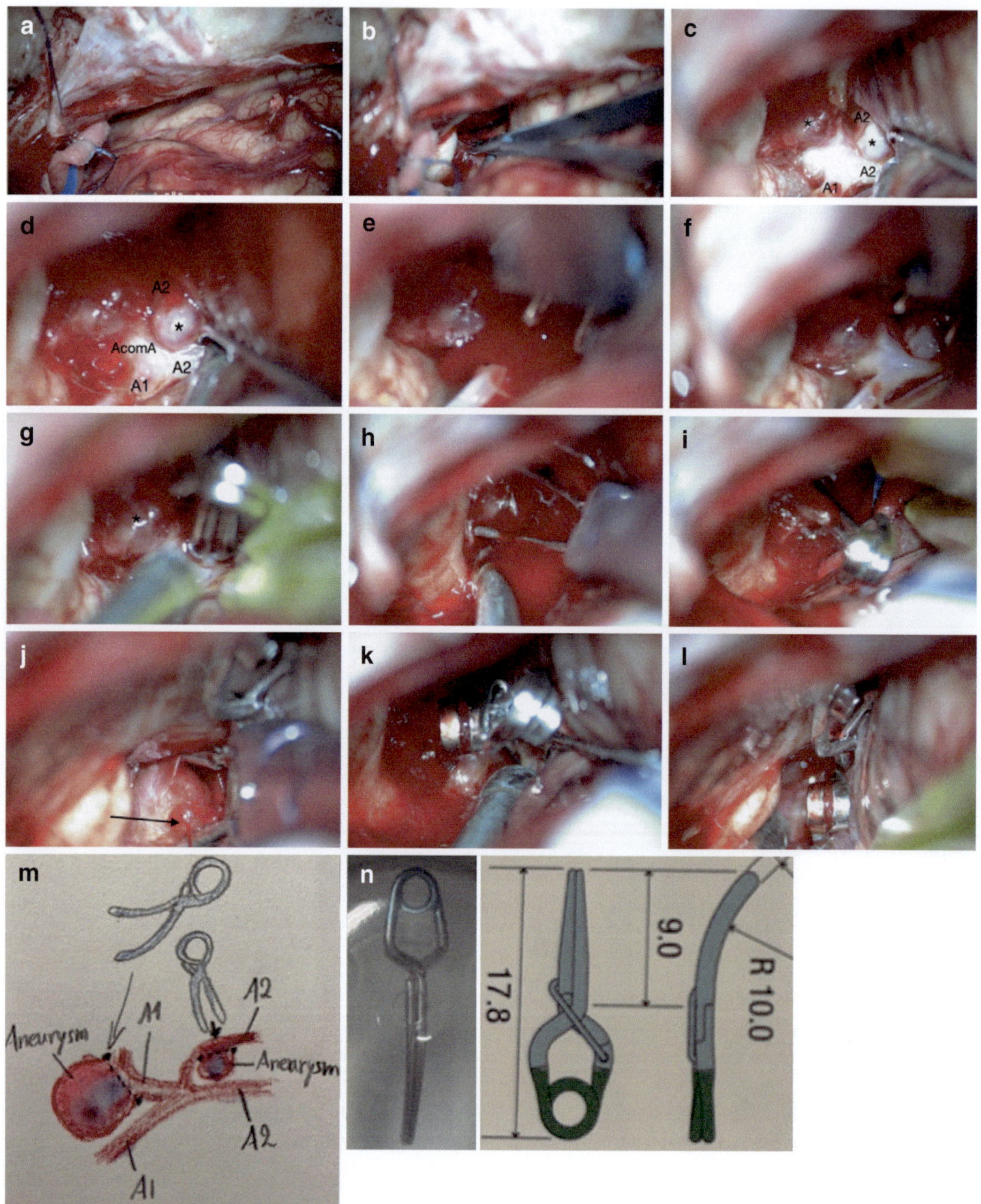

Fig. 7.23 Microsurgical aneurysm clipping of the patient with an A1-A2 aneurysm left and a proximal A2 aneurysm right (illustrated in Fig. 7.20). We choose a right subfrontal approach to clip the aneurysms, to avoid the dominant brain hemisphere. (**a**) Subfrontal approach. The retroflexion of the head together with CSF drainage forms already a spontaneous corridor between brain and skull base, rendering the use of retractors obsolete. (**b**) Sharp dissection to open the basal cisterns and identify the optic nerve and the carotid cisterns. (**c**) Both aneurysms can be seen (asterisk: aneurysms). (**d**) The A2 aneurysm (asterisk) is dissected. (**e**) In the attempt to clip the aneurysm and only with the slightest manipulation, the aneurysm ruptured intraoperatively. (**f**) Pilot clip application in the intraoperatively ruptured A2 aneurysm. (**g**) Cessation of the bleeding after clip application of a bayonetted clip, which is not disturbing the further dissection of the second aneurysm (asterisk). (**h**) The second aneurysm (which had a very thin wall) ruptured too and a curved pilot clip was placed to this one too. (**i**) After pilot clip application to the A1-A2 aneurysm, we dissected the aneurysm and (**j**) replaced the clip (the arrow shows the bleeding point of the aneurysm). (**k**) The A1-A2 aneurysm is clipped after repositioning the clip. (**l**) The A2 aneurysm is permanently clipped to be a curved clip. (**m**) Schematic drawing of the operation. (**n**) The clip used to occlude the aneurysms. Slightly curved clip (2×)

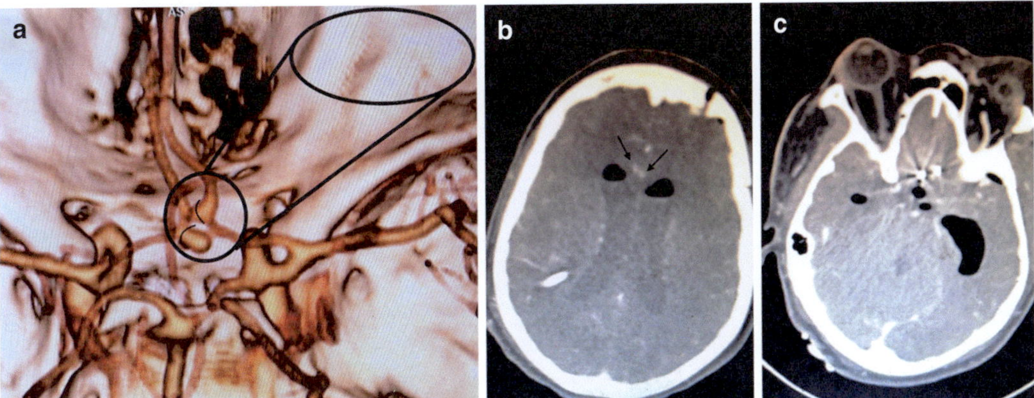

Fig. 7.24 Postoperative CTA of the patient with an A1-A2 aneurysm left and a proximal A2 aneurysm right. (**a**) The cone illustrates the surgical corridor and the black lines on the aneurysms the position of the clips. (**b**) The CTA shows perfused A2 on both hemispheres (arrows). (**c**) The clips are seen, and as far as possible (caused by artifacts), no aneurysms can be detected

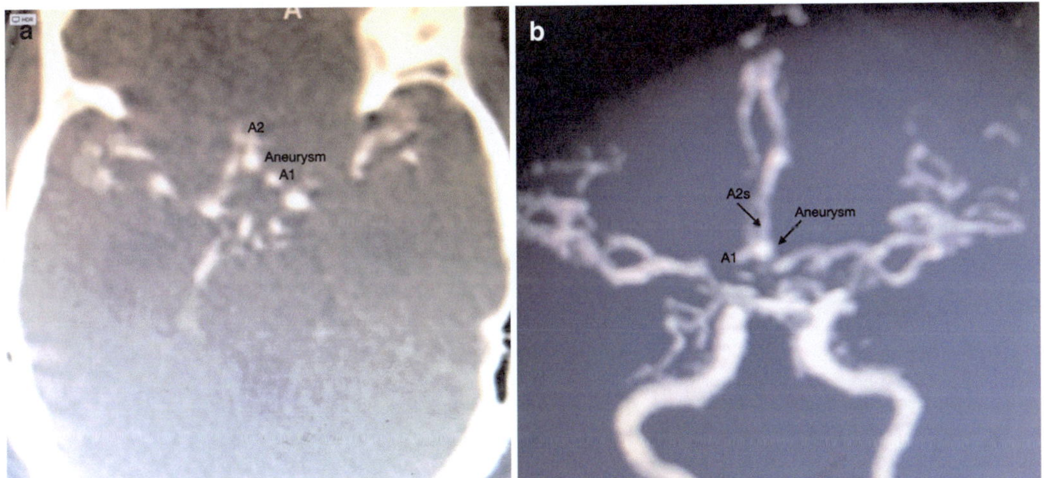

Fig. 7.25 Complex left AcomA aneurysm adhering to the frontopolar and right A1 artery in a 56-year-old male patient with SAH due to ruptured AcomA aneurysm. (**a**) CTA showing an AcomA aneurysm. (**b**) CTA 3D reconstruction showing that the aneurysm is located frontal of the AcomA

the dissection of the carotid and A1, leading us to the aneurysm. As depicted in Fig. 7.29, the aneurysm was adhered to the brain tissue, presenting a challenge for dissection, albeit achievable using a blunt dissector. Both sides' A2s were identified along with the aneurysm neck. Upon complete dissection of the neck, a clear perspective for clip placement was obtained, and the aneurysm was secured using a 9-mm straight clip, a standard clip available in our basic clip inventory. Notably, our armamentarium doesn't include 5 mm clips.

We adapt by using 9-mm clips even if shorter lengths might suffice. In instances where shorter clips are necessary, we adjust the depth of clipping based on the aneurysm's neck size. Working with longer-bladed clips emphasizes the need to ensure that the A2s are positioned away from the clip blades and that the aneurysm is fully occluded. Thorough inspection to assure perfusion of both A2s is essential. Dissection of the A2 can be time-consuming, often requiring approximately 30 min more, especially in cases involving adhesions.

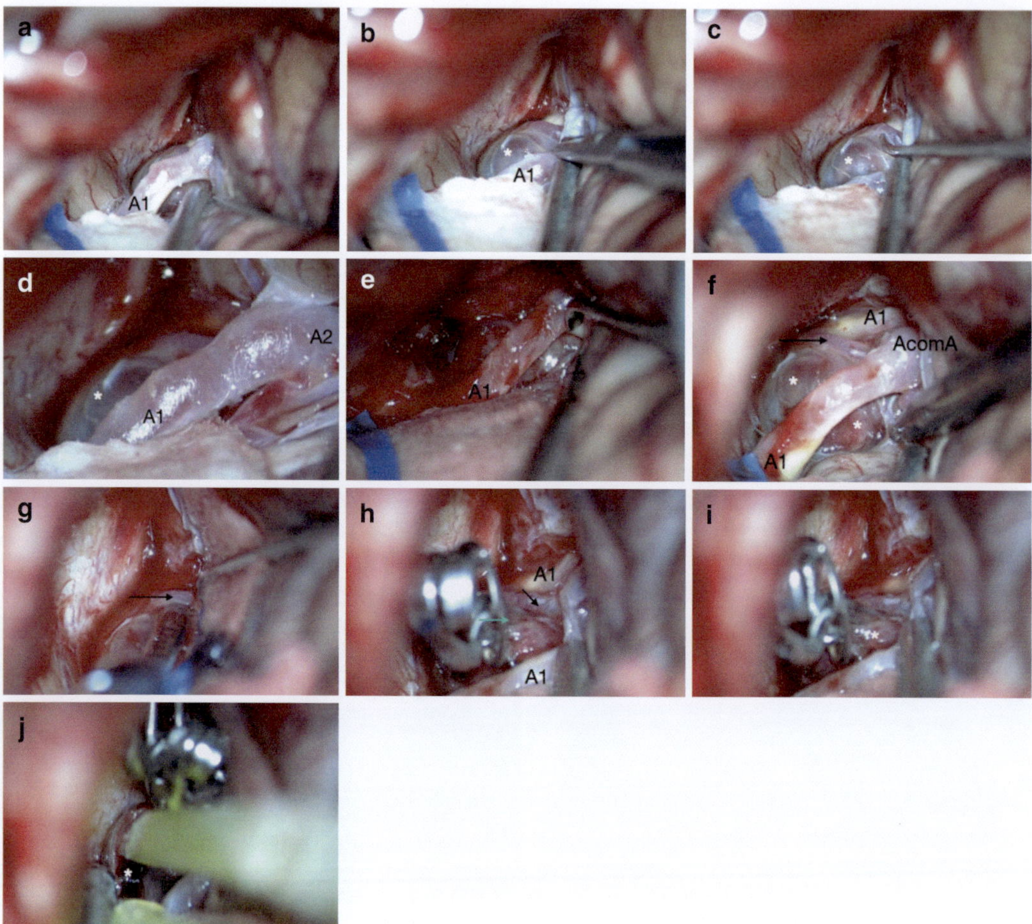

Fig. 7.26 Microsurgical clipping of a complex left AcomA aneurysm adhering to the frontopolar and right A1 artery (see Fig. 7.25). (**a**) Subfrontal approach and following the A1 toward the AcomA complex. (**b**) Approaching the AcomA the aneurysm can be seen (white asterisk). The inferior side of A1 is adhering to the aneurysm. (**c**) The frontopolar artery is adherent to the aneurysm (asterisk) and had to be dissected free from the aneurysm wall in order to pass a clip under the artery and prevent occlusion of the vessel. The microdissector is placed between the artery and the aneurysm heading away from the aneurysm in order to prevent its rupture. (**d**) Aneurysm (asterisk), A1 and A2 junction ipsilateral is seen. (**e**) The aneurysm (asterisk) is inspected anterior and posterior to the ipsilateral A1. (**f**) Dissection of the neck proceeds carefully in order to define the aneurysm neck (asterisk shows the aneurysm anterior and posterior to the A1). The AcomA and the contralateral A1 are identified. The contralateral A1 is adhering to the aneurysm wall too. The arrow indicates the frontopolar artery, which was adhering to the aneurysm wall. (**g**) Placing the straight 9 mm aneurysm clip between the aneurysm and the dissected frontopolar artery (arrow). The A1 was also dissected and is not included in the clip; therefore, its perfusion is not disturbed. (**h**) The aneurysm is clipped, and both A1s and the frontopolar artery (black arrow) are free and not in the clip blades. A small dog ear (blue arrow) is left. (**i**) The dog ear (asterisk) is clipped by a mini aneurysm clip. (**j**) The aneurysm is widely opened (asterisk), and thrombotic material is removed

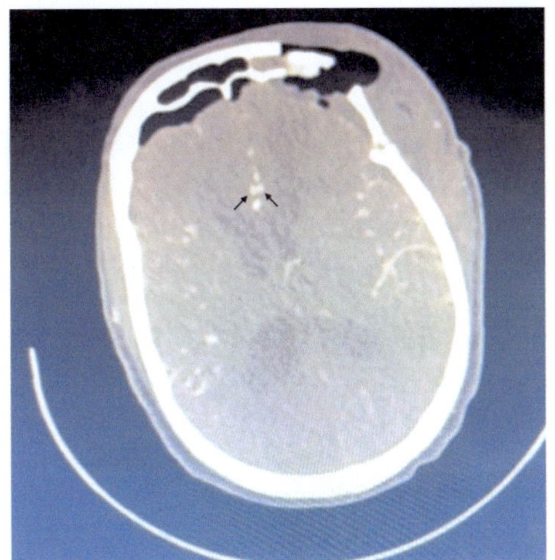

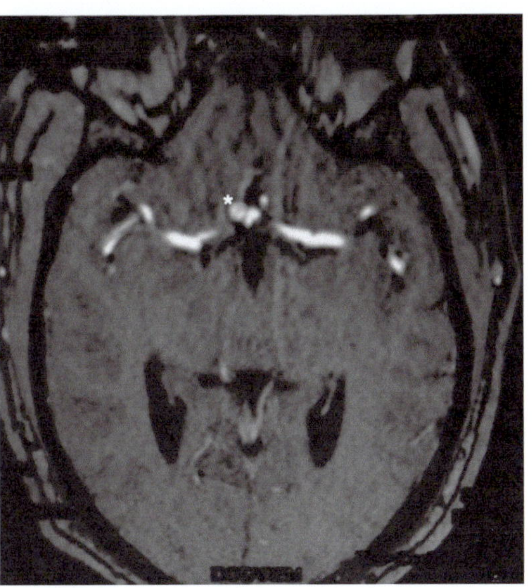

Fig. 7.27 Postoperative imaging of the clipped complex left AcomA aneurysm (Figs. 7.25 and 7.26). In a case like this, where the arteries are extremely adherent to the aneurysm, it is important to control perfusion of the A2s on both sides in the postoperative CTA. Both A2s are perfused (black arrows). The occlusion of the aneurysm was controlled intraoperatively by opening the aneurysm sack. The frontal sinus was opened during the craniotomy and was closed by a muscle patch pushed in the ostium. Before that, the mucosa of the frontal sinus was coagulated in order to prevent a mucocele in the long term

Fig. 7.28 MRA shows an AcomA aneurysm (asterisk) in a 48-year-old male patient who suffered an SAH 3 months ago

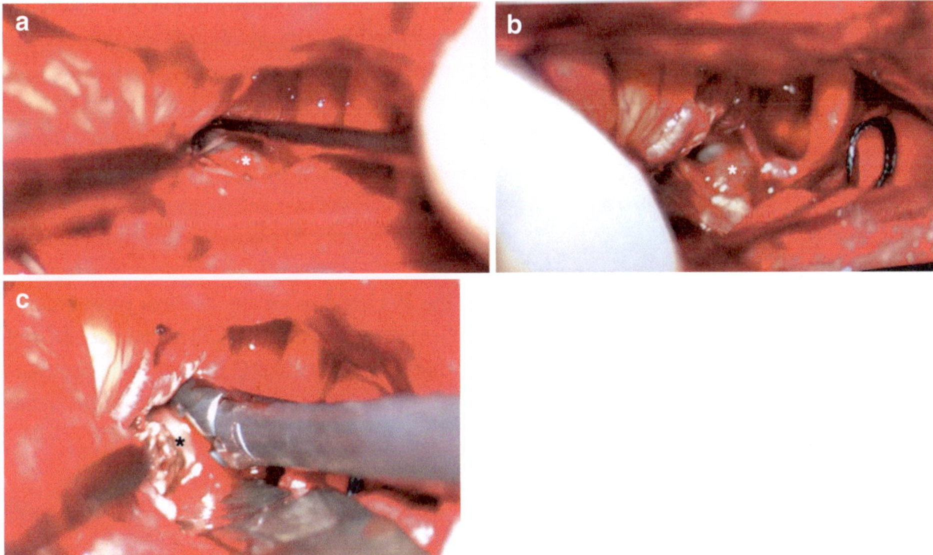

Fig. 7.29 Microsurgical clipping of ruptured AcomA aneurysm (see Fig. 7.28). (**a**) The aneurysm (white asterisk) is surrounded by thick arachnoid tissue, which is difficult to remove in order to dissect the aneurysm free. The arachnoid is sticking on the aneurysm wall, and sharp dissection is dangerous, since it can lead to aneurysm rupture, but blunt dissection is dangerous too. (**b**) Very careful sharp dissection allowed us to remove part of the arachnoid tissue in order to identify parts of the aneurysm (white asterisk) and to follow the sack toward the neck. (**c**) After identifying the neck, we left a small tissue bridge of arachnoid (black asterisk) on the aneurysm and clipped the aneurysm (arachnoid tissue including)

7.4 Clipping of Pericallosal Artery Aneurysms

Pericallosal arterie aneurysms can pose challenges in localising them. In many cases in the Western world, neuronavigation is utilized for such aneurysms; however, this technology is unavailable in low-income countries. A 45-year-old man experienced a WFNS grade 4 SAH caused by a pericallosal aneurysm, as revealed in the CTA performed 2 months ago (Fig. 7.30). An initial attempt to clip the aneurysm failed due to difficulty in localizing it, resulting in the clip being placed approximately 2 cm proximal to the aneurysm. A second attempt was planned during the vascular expert's visit with the objective of successfully clipping the aneurysm and providing guidance on preventing failures in pericallosal artery aneurysm clipping.

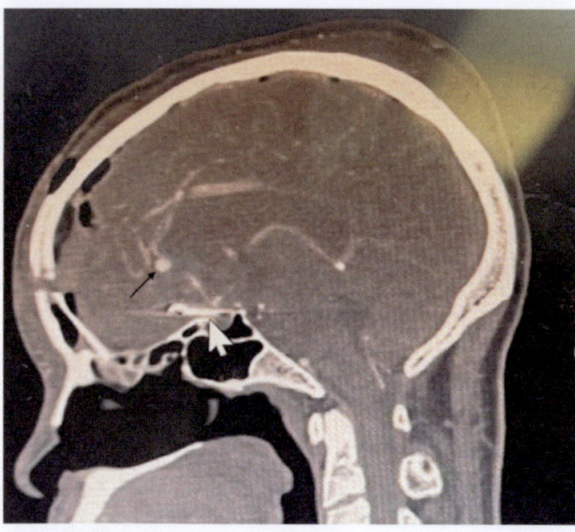

Fig. 7.30 A 45-year-old man suffered a WFNS grade 4 SAH, caused by a pericallosal aneurysm. Sagittal CTA reconstruction showing a pericallosal artery aneurysm in a previously operated patient where the aneurysm was missed. The black arrow indicates the aneurysm and the white arrow the previously placed clip of the first surgery

Given the absence of neuronavigation, identifying vascular anatomy intraoperatively became pivotal. The aneurysm stemmed from the bifurcation of the pericallosal and callosomarginal arteries, serving as crucial anatomical landmarks for intraoperative identification.

The previous craniotomy was reopened and extended toward the frontal bone. We proceeded interhemispherically, following the path illustrated in Fig. 7.31, toward the callosomarginal artery and successfully identified the vessel along with both pericallosal arteries. At this stage, the aneurysm remained concealed within scar tissue and was not manipulated or touched. Subsequently, the previous clip was located, and dissection around the clip aided in identifying the proximal A2, enabling proximal control if necessary. Further dissection of the aneurysm ensued, requiring the liberation of the callosomarginal artery that adhered to the aneurysm wall. It took considerable time to discern the aneurysm neck and liberate the callosomarginal artery.

A safe corridor for clipping without jeopardizing nearby vessels is paramount. The aneurysm was clipped according to the guidance provided in Fig. 7.31 and subsequently opened to eliminate thrombotic material, ensuring complete occlusion, and overseeing the status of the neighboring vessels. As a final step, we examined the previously placed clip from the initial operation, but opted against its removal, considering the proximity of small vessels that might be inadvertently damaged. The patient was transferred to the ICU and extubated 2 days postsurgery, given his presurgical GCS of 11. Despite this, an immediate postoperative CTA was conducted to evaluate the perfusion status of adjacent vessels (as depicted in Fig. 7.32).

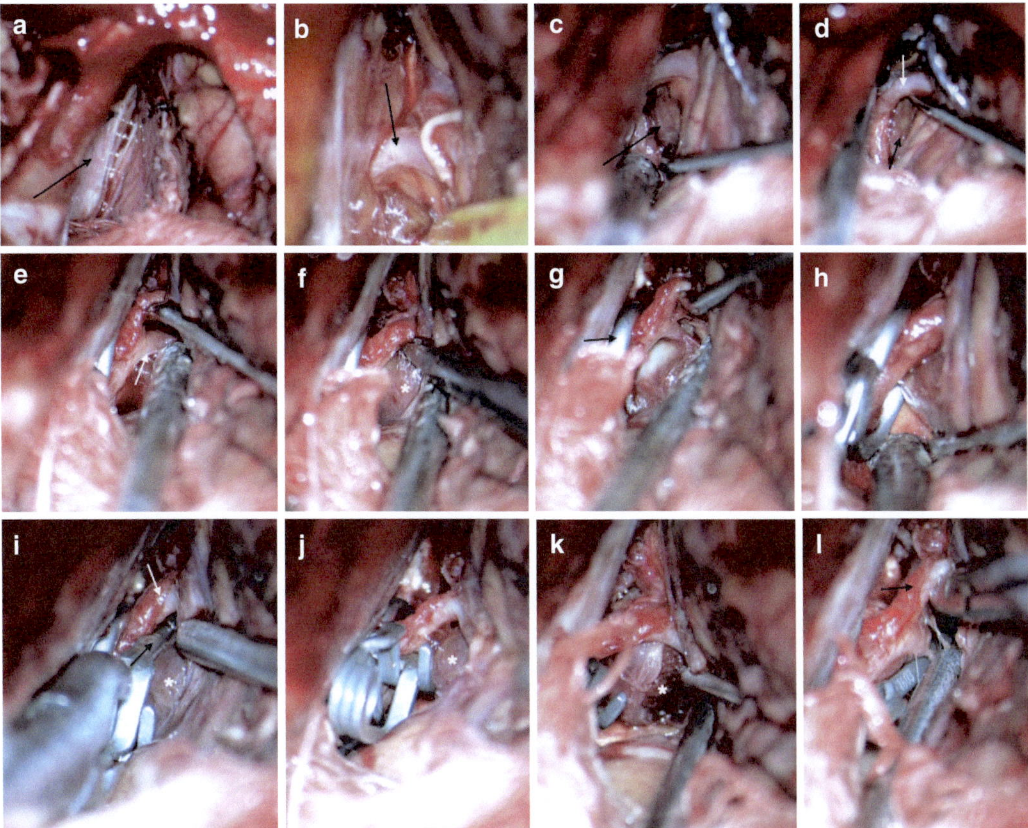

Fig. 7.31 Clipping of the pericallosal artery aneurysm seen in Fig. 7.30. (**a**) Interhemispheric approach to identify the callosomarginal artery as a first step. The arrow indicates the falx. (**b**) The callosomarginal artery (black arrow) is identified. (**c**) The aneurysm (black arrow) is palpated and visualized under a layer of arachnoid scar tissue. (**d**) Further dissection shows adherence of the callosomarginal artery to the aneurysm. It was still not clear where the aneurysm originates from. (**e**) The callosomarginal artery is dissected free from the aneurysm, which is still covered by a thin scar tissue layer (white arrow). (**f**) Removal of the scar tissue from the aneurysm (asterisk) in order to define the aneurysm sack and follow it to its neck. (**g**) The aneurysm is clipped at first with a fenestrated straight pilot clip (black arrow). The callosomarginal artery is in the fenestration of the clip. (**h**) The aneurysm is clipped at first, and now we proceed with further dissection around the aneurysm sack. (**i**) Further dissection of the aneurysm allows a better visualization of the neck, and now a straight clip was used in front of the callosomarginal artery as seen in the picture. The black arrow indicates the direction of the clip blade and the white arrow the freed callosomarginal artery. (**j**) The aneurysm (white asterisk) is safely clipped, and the fenestrated clip, which is still on place, will be removed now. (**k**) The aneurysm is opened widely, and thrombotic material is removed in order to (**l**) see around the aneurysm and exclude the possibility of occlusion of any artery around the clip

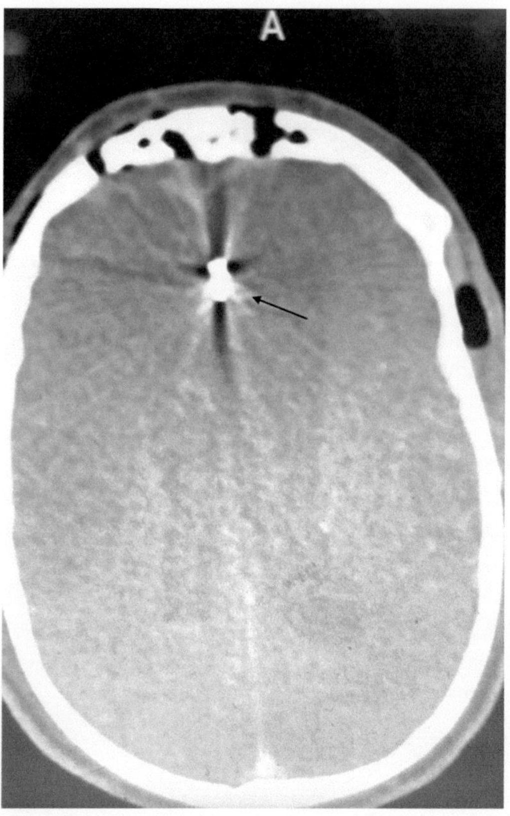

Fig. 7.32 Postsurgical CTA of the clipping shown in Fig. 7.31. The CTA shows an intact pericallosal artery close to the clip (black arrow). The native CT, which is not shown, has no signs of infarctions

7.5 Extradural, Cavernous Sinus Segment Symptomatic Fusiform Aneurysms

During our fellowship program in Cameroon and Tanzania, we opted to perform occlusions on extradural cavernous sinus aneurysms in three patients (two in Cameroon and one in Tanzania). In Western medical practice, the preferred treatment approach for such aneurysms typically involves stent placement, but this option was not feasible in our circumstances. Given that the aneurysms were thrombotic and led to ischemic episodes in the patients, we determined that occluding the aneurysm was warranted.

Our plan for all three patients involved occluding the internal carotid artery (ICA) distal to the aneurysm to induce thrombosis in both the aneu-

rysm and the ICA. For the two patients in Cameroon, we conducted the occlusion distal to the aneurysm in an awake surgery setting. However, in the case of the third patient in Tanzania, prior to ICA occlusion, a carotid artery (ECA)—saphenous vein—M3 high-flow bypass was performed. The micro-instruments necessary for this bypass procedure were brought by the expert surgeon himself, carrying his portable set from country to country.

7.5.1 ICA Occlusion in Awake Surgery

There were two cases of thrombotic aneurysms of the cavernous sinus segment of the carotid artery in Cameroon, necessitating occlusion of the internal carotid artery (ICA) distal to the aneurysms (Fig. 7.33). Given the limited resources at our disposal, this endeavor was particularly challenging. We grappled with how to ensure that clip occlusion of the carotid wouldn't result in carotid infarction and consequential devastating outcomes in the brain. Unfortunately, we didn't have the necessary equipment at that time to perform a high-flow bypass or any bypass within the brain, so we needed to explore alternative solutions.

We opted for a two-step surgical approach. In the initial surgery, the patient was under full anesthesia, and we surgically exposed and dissected the internal carotid artery (ICA) to precisely locate the site where the clip should be placed to occlude it (Fig. 7.34), as relying solely on a presurgical manual occlusion of the carotid isn't sufficiently reliable or safe for performing an ICA occlusion (the test showed no neurological deficits), we then replaced the bone and closed the wound and choose to clip-occlude the artery in a second awake surgical procedure.

Subsequently, 2–3 days after the first surgery, a second procedure was planned under local anesthesia, while the patients were fully awake. We reopened the wound and accessed the previously dissected ICA. We proceeded with the ICA occlusion and requested the patients to move their extremities at 45-s intervals until the wound clo-

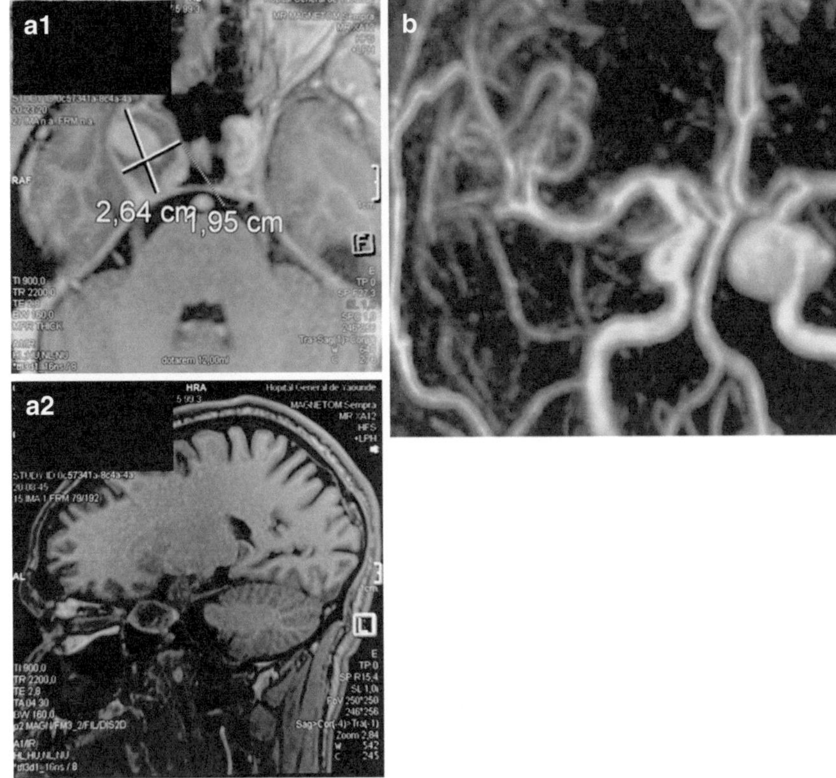

Fig. 7.33 Extradural ICA aneurysm of the cavernous sinus of two patients. These aneurysms caused diplopia, and under the suspicion of aneurysm growth, action was needed. (**a1**) MRA (transverse section) showing a partially thrombosed aneurysm in the right ICA of the cavernous sinus in patient 1. (**a2**) Sagittal section of T1-weighted MRI shows the location of the aneurysm. (**b**) MRA 3D reconstruction of the intracranial arteries showing the aneurysm in the left ICA in patient 2

sure. Subsequently, we closely monitored the patients' neurological status in the ICU for the initial 48 h. The patients exhibited satisfactory collateral perfusion, and postoperative CTAs revealed no signs of infarctions. There was a robust signal from all intracerebral vessels, and a complete thrombosis of the occluded ICA (Fig. 7.35).

Both patients were discharged home in good condition 1 week after surgery. The male patient experienced no deficits. However, the other patient (female) encountered transient ischemic attacks (TIAs). After consulting the local vascular expert team in Cameroon, it was determined that a high-flow bypass should be performed during the next visit. The necessary equipment was provided by charitable sponsors and subsequently carried as personal equipment by the expert sur-

geon during visits to various countries as mentioned above.

Preoperatively, a native CCT scan was conducted, revealing small infarctions in the affected hemisphere. These infarctions were likely due to hypotensive episodes, resulting in compromised perfusion in the hemisphere. This led to the development of small infarcts, causing hemiparesis, speech problems, and vision disturbances in the female patient. In her third surgery, a high-flow common carotid artery (CCA)—saphenous vein—M2 middle cerebral artery (MCA) bypass was performed to restore blood flow to the affected hemisphere and prevent further ischemic episodes. Following the bypass procedure, the neurological condition of the patient began to improve.

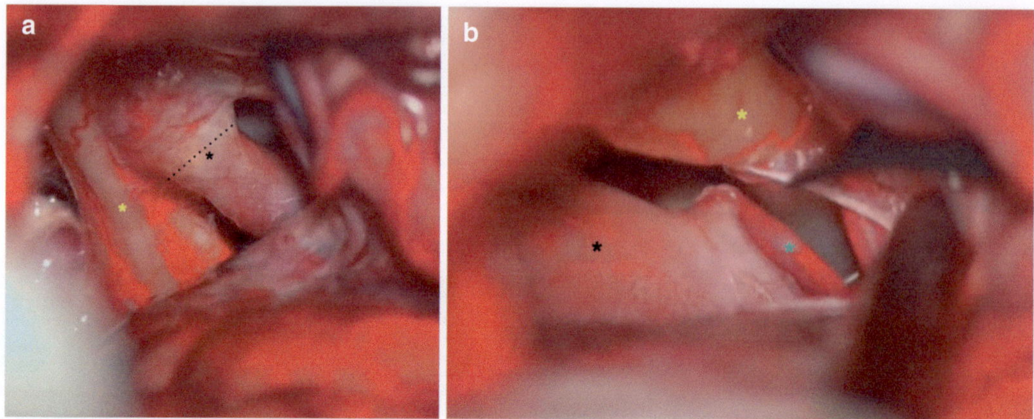

Fig. 7.34 Occlusion of the ICA in patient 1 (Fig. 7.33). In a first surgery, the patient was under full anesthesia, and the ICA dissected free in order to identify the localization where the clip should be placed to occlude the ICA in a later surgery, where the patient was awake in order to control for any deficits. (**a**) Subfrontal approach to the optic nerve and the intradural carotid (asterisk). The dotted line shows the position where the aneurysm clip will be placed in the second surgery, which will be performed in 2–3 days. (**b**) Carotid (black asterisk) and pcoma are identified. The clip has to be placed proximal to the pcoma in order to prevent any pcoma infarction. Right of the carotid (white asterisk) is the oculomotor nerve

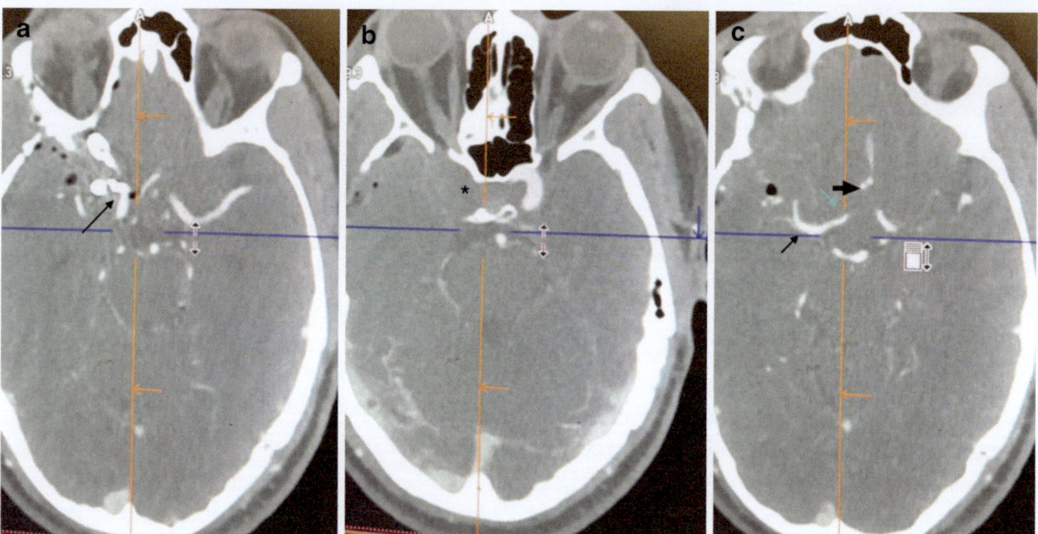

Fig. 7.35 CTA 2 days after occlusion of the intradural ICA (patient 1 of Fig. 7.33). (**a**) Distal to the clip (black arrow), the carotid shows a satisfying perfusion. (**b**) Proximal to the clip, there is no carotid artery signal (asterisk) indicating the thrombosed artery, which also leads to aneurysm thrombosis. The left ICA has a physiologic signal. (**c**) After clip occlusion of the right ICA the M1 of the right side (black thin arrow), the right A1 (blue arrow) and the A2 (thick black arrow) are all perfused indicating an excellent perfusion from the contralateral ICA

7.5.2 High-Flow, Carotid-Saphenous Vein-MCA, Bypass

We conducted two high-flow bypass surgical procedures during the fellowship programs. One of these procedures involved the patient discussed in Sect. 7.5.1, while the other involved a male patient in Tanzania who experienced transient ischemic attack (TIA) episodes in the affected hemispheres due to an extradural cavernous segment thrombotic aneurysm. Both bypass surgeries followed the typical approach outlined in the existing literature. However, we will outline the primary steps of this surgery for the purpose of education.

The surgery was conducted collaboratively, employing an interdisciplinary approach involving vascular surgeons. The saphenous vein (25 cm) was harvested by the vascular surgeon, who also performed dissection of the carotid artery in the neck, specifically involving the common carotid artery (CCA), external carotid artery (ECA), and internal carotid artery (ICA) complex.

The harvested saphenous vein was placed in a heparin bath and thoroughly rinsed with heparin solution. To ensure proper directional placement of the bypass, the vein was marked for directionality from proximal to distal. This directional marking is crucial due to the presence of valves in the vein. It signifies that the distal end of the saphenous vein should be anastomosed to the carotid in the neck, while the proximal end connects to the cerebral vessel.

Subsequently, the vein was tunneled subcutaneously anterior to the ear, and a pterional craniotomy was performed. Opening the Sylvian fissure enabled identification of a suitable MCA branch artery (M2 or M3). Initially, we conducted the ECA-saphenous vein anastomosis using 7-0 nonabsorbable suture material. The anastomosed vein was clip-occluded close to the carotid artery to prevent thrombosis resulting from blood stasis. Following this, the distal anastomosis (saphenous vein to M3 in one case and M2 in the other) was

established. Notably, the patients did not receive heparinization during this procedure.

In the male patient (46 years old), the bypass appeared nonpulsatile, and upon temporary occlusion of the intracranial intradural ICA, immediate brain edema occurred, signifying both the bypass's critical need and its probable lack of integrity. Upon removing the temporary clip from the intracranial ICA, we meticulously examined the bypass for potential thrombosis. A small thrombus was identified in the proximal part of the bypass (ECA-saphenous vein).

To address this, we carefully opened the saphenous vein with a straight 5-mm cut beyond the thrombus, maneuvering the thrombus into the ECA and thoroughly rinsed the vessels with a heparin solution. The vein was subsequently repaired using two single stitches. Following these interventions, the bypass exhibited full functionality and pulsation.

With assured bypass integrity, a second attempt to occlude the ICA distal to the aneurysm was successful without any observed brain edema. The surgical site was closed, and the patient was extubated in the operating room. Upon transfer to the ICU, the patient remained neurologically intact. Please refer to Fig. 7.36 for a visual depiction of the surgical procedure.

7.5.3 Outcome of the High-Flow Bypass Procedures

Two high-flow bypass surgeries were carried out as previously described in Sect. 7.5. Throughout the intraoperative phase, the bypasses appeared functionally sound and intact. In the case of the female patient from Cameroon, who encountered a perfusion deficit following occlusion of the internal carotid artery (ICA) and subsequently underwent a high-flow bypass procedure, notable improvements were observed in her neurological symptoms. Additionally, the manual occlusion test conducted on the unaffected ICA exhibited no resulting deficits, indicating the successful functionality of the bypass. This positive outcome implied sufficient perfusion to both cerebral hemispheres, affirming the efficacy of the bypass in restoring circulation.

However, the aftermath of the second case was more intricate. In the case involving the 46-year-old male patient from Tanzania, as previously detailed in Sect. 7.5.2, the immediate postsurgery period showed promising signs. Upon transfer to the intensive care unit (ICU), the patient demonstrated favorable neurological indicators, exhibiting movement in all four extremities. Unfortunately, around 3 h after the surgical intervention, he developed a subcutaneous hematoma on the head, prompting contralateral hemiparesis and raising concerns about potential compression affecting the bypass. A rapid response ensued, facilitating the patient's swift transfer back to the operating room. There, a surgical procedure was performed to remove the hematoma. Subsequent examination of the bypass after hematoma removal concluded that the hematoma did not result from any bypass-related leakage or issues associated with the vein used for the bypass. Further scrutiny affirmed that the bypass was fully functional, indicating its integrity and continuous pulsatile flow.

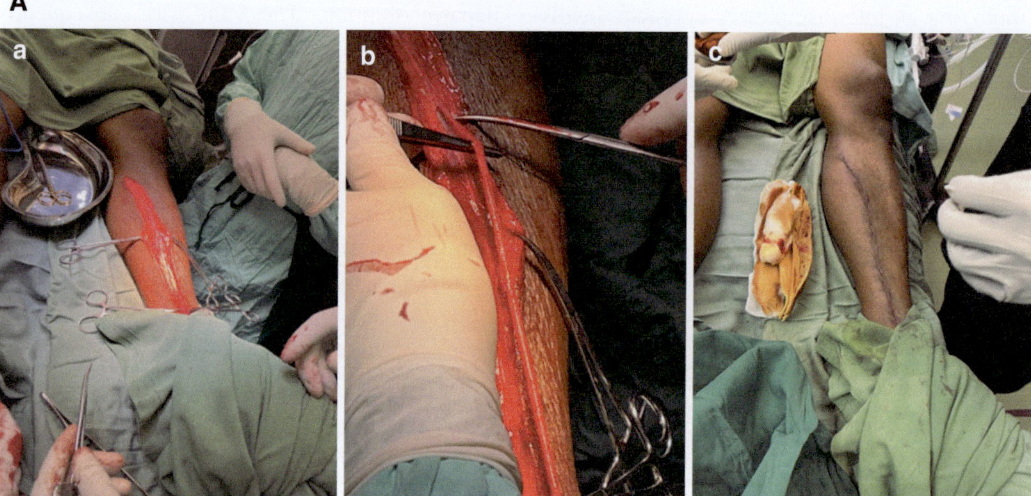

Fig. 7.36 (**A**) Harvesting the saphenous vein for high flow EC-IC bypass. (**a**) A long cut over the saphenous vein was performed in order to harvest about 25 cm. The surgery was performed by the vascular surgeon in an interdisciplinary approach. (**b**) Close up of the dissected vein. (**c**) Skin closure after harvesting the saphenous vein. (**B**) High flow ECA-saphenous vein-M3 MCA bypass. The harvested saphenous vein will be anastomosed to the ECA and then on the M3 MCA artery to establish a bypass and safely occlude the ipsilateral ICA in order to reach thrombosis of a cavernous segment ICA aneurysm. (**a**) After dissection of the ECA (black asterisk) by the vascular surgeon, temporary clip occlusion of the proximal and distal part of the ECA as well as its branches was performed. The dotted line shows the planed carotidectomy. The blue asterisk indicates the saphenous vein, which will be anastomosed. The direction of the saphenous vein is distal end anastomosed to the ECA and proximal end to the M3. (**b**) First stitch is placed to approximate the saphenous vein to the carotid artery. (**c**) Proceeding with the anastomosis on one side with single suturing. (**d**) Suturing the other side of the saphenous vein (black asterisk). (**e**) After pterional craniotomy, the proximal end of the saphenous (asterisk) will be sutured in the dissected M3 (double asterisk). The M3 is cut open longitudinally in order to place the anastomosis. (**f**) Suturing the saphenous vein (asterisk) to the M3 (double asterisk) in a continuous fashion. (**g**) Proceeding the anastomosis (asterisk) on the opposite side. (**h**) Removing the temporary clips from the distal M3 and the proximal M3. Some significant bleeding from the anastomosis is repaired by single stitches (asterisk: saphenous vein). (**i**) After removing the temporary clip from the proximal M3 again, no leakage bleeding is seen, and the saphenous vein (asterisk) is filled immediately. Removal of the temporary clip of the saphenous vein close to the ECA leads to a good pulsation of the vein

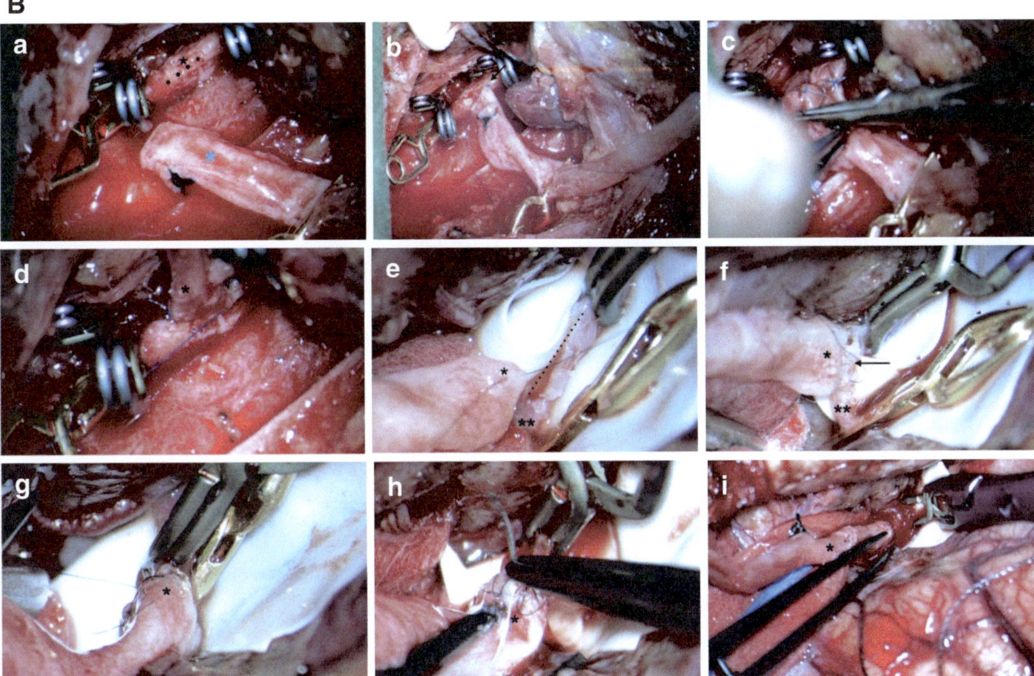

Fig. 7.36 (continued)

7.6 Explorative Surgery in Cases with CTA-Negative Subarachnoid Hemorrhage

In four cases, patients presented with a subarachnoid hemorrhage (SAH) characterized by extensive bleeding within the basal cisterns, classified as Fisher grade 4. Despite conducting a comprehensive examination via CT angiography (CTA), no detectable aneurysms were observed. It's imperative to note that CT scans have limitations in detecting aneurysms smaller than 2 mm, and in low-income countries, access to angiography, a more precise diagnostic tool, is often limited or unavailable.

Given the absence of identified aneurysms in the CTA, exploratory craniotomy and direct visual inspection of the cerebral vessels became a viable approach for these cases. The craniotomy was strategically performed on the side exhibiting more extensive blood accumulation. A classical pterional craniotomy was executed, allowing meticulous dissection of the cerebral vessels in a proximal to distal fashion. This method was adopted to establish proximal control if an aneurysm, which might not have been localized at the initial examination, was to rupture prematurely during the exploration.

The meticulous dissection commenced with the internal carotid artery (ICA), followed by the ophthalmic artery, posterior communicating artery (pcomA), the first segment of the middle cerebral artery (M1), the M1-M2 bifurcation, the A1 segments of the anterior cerebral artery (A1s), the anterior communicating artery (AcomA), the ICA on the contralateral side, the A1-A2 segments on the ipsilateral side, and the A1-A2 segments on the contralateral side. The dissection then proceeded with the meticulous opening of the Lilliequist membrane, allowing for visualization and inspection of the basilar tip and basilar artery, preferably from the carotid-oculomotor triangle.

Extreme caution was exercised throughout the process to avoid inadvertent manipulation of a potential blister aneurysm that could lead to its rupture without having established proximal vascular control or elucidated the aneurysm's anatomy and precise location.

Remarkably, in one of the four cases, an ophthalmic artery aneurysm was successfully identified and clipped during the exploration, despite not being visualized in the initial CTA after the SAH. This emphasized the significance of direct surgical exploration in cases where conventional diagnostic imaging methods might fail to detect certain aneurysms.

7.7　Arteriovenous Malformations (AVM) of the Brain

7.7.1　AVM of the Left Lateral Ventricle

A 25-year-old mathematics student has been experiencing recurrent seizures and intraventricular bleedings over the past few years. Upon conducting a computed tomography angiography (CTA), an arteriovenous malformation (AVM) located in the left lateral ventricle was identified (refer to Fig. 7.37). However, due to the static nature of the CTA image, the precise identification of feeders and draining veins associated with the AVM necessitated intraoperative determination.

Considering the recurring bleedings, the decision to surgically remove the AVM was made. Fortunately, the AVM's location within the left ventricle allowed for navigational access, even without the availability of neuronavigation tools. An incision was made over the midline, with a craniotomy measuring 1/3 (2 cm) on the right and 2/3 (4 cm) on the left side of the superior sagittal sinus (SSS). Subsequently, the dura on the left side was opened toward the SSS to access the ventricle.

Using a cannula, the left ventricle was punctured through the Koher's point, allowing for the controlled release of cerebrospinal fluid (CSF) (as depicted in Fig. 7.38). Further dissection around the canal was meticulously conducted until reaching the ventricle. Upon opening the ventricle, the AVM became visible, necessitating the use of retractors for better visualization.

Precise identification of the AVM's anatomy and differentiation between feeding arteries and draining veins were achieved through meticulous dissection and temporary clipping of the vessels. Whenever a temporarily occluded vessel was suspected to be a vein, the clip was removed to prevent AVM rupture. Conversely, if the occluded vessel was identified as an artery, the clip remained in place, allowing continued dissection of the AVM. Once the AVM dissection was completed, all identified feeder vessels were coagulated, and the AVM was successfully excised.

Key aspects of this surgical procedure are illustrated in Fig. 7.39, while the postsurgical outcome is depicted in Fig. 7.40. This comprehensive approach ensured the safe and effective removal of the AVM, mitigating the risk of recurrent bleedings and improving the patient's prognosis.

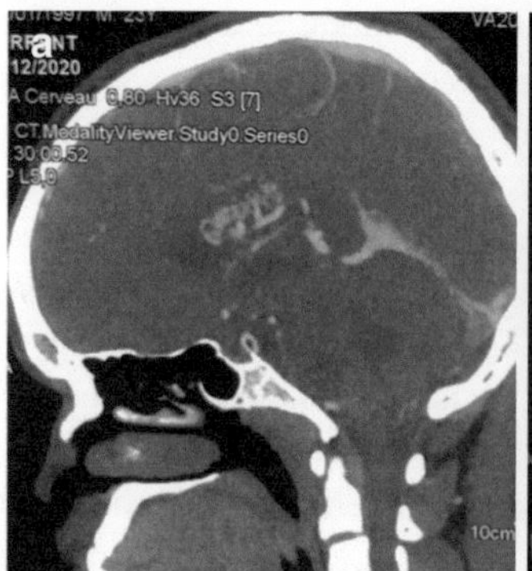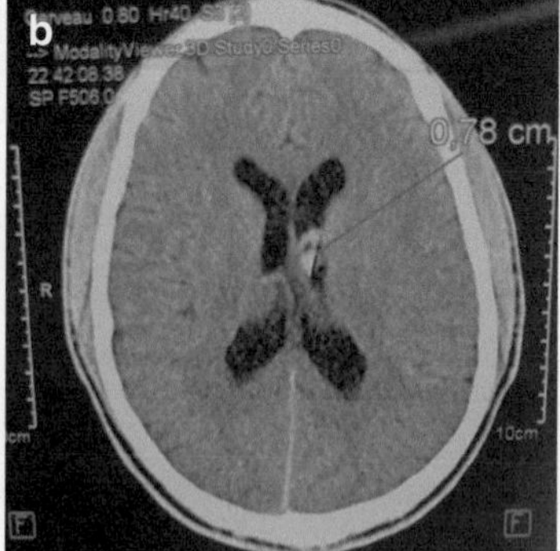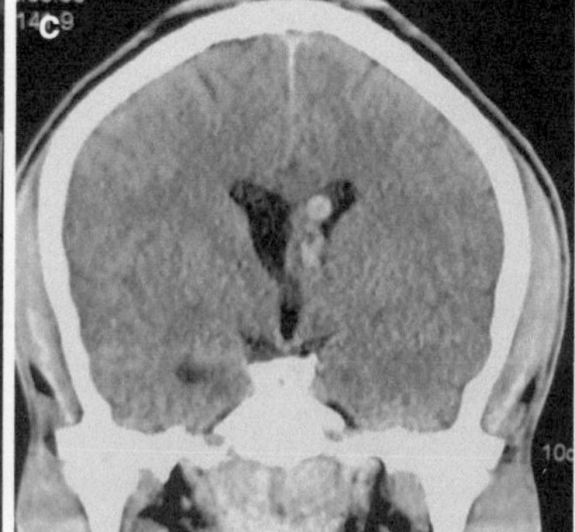

Fig. 7.37 CTA of a 25-year-old male with intraventricular AVM. (**a**) Sagittal CTA reconstruction showing the intraventricular AVM. (**b**) In this native cranial CT, there is some bleeding around the AVM indicating leakage. (**c**) Coronal reconstruction of the cranial CT with the AVM in the left ventricle

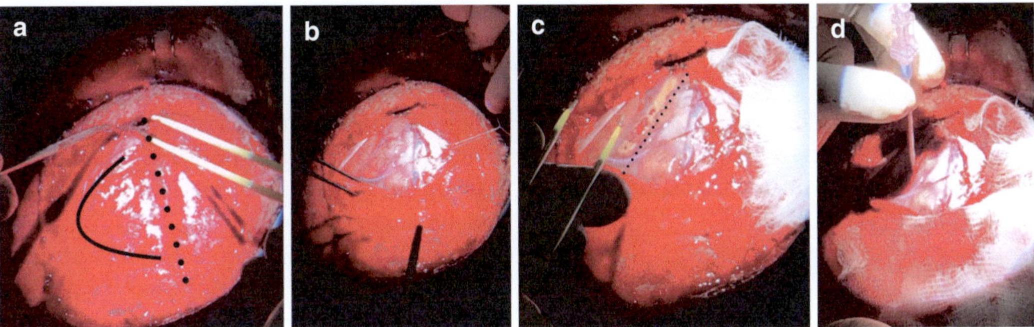

Fig. 7.38 Approaching the intraventricular AVM. (**a**) Midline skin cut and craniotomy focused on 11 cm over the midpupillary line (dotted line, superior sagittal sinus; curved line, planned dura opening center over Kocher's point). (**b**) The dura is opened with its base toward the superior sagittal sinus. (**c**) Cortical bipolar coagulation over Kocher's point and in a length of 2 cm (dotted line). (**d**) Placing a ventricular catheter to the lateral ventricle in order to use this projection to proceed to the AVM

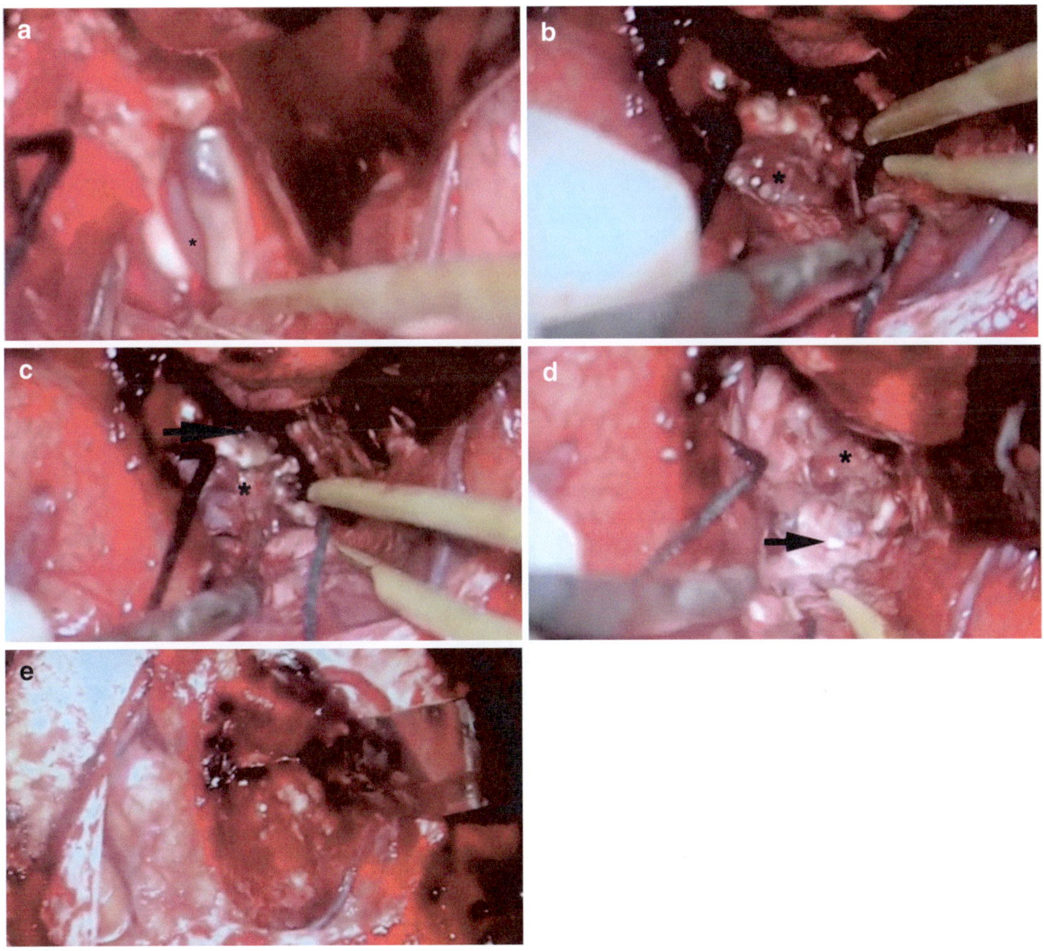

Fig. 7.39 Microsurgical removal of the intraventricular AVM (see Fig. 7.37). (**a**) After following the ventricular catheter to the ventricle, we opened the ventricle and identified the arterialized vein (asterisk). (**b**) Careful dissection around the AVM (asterisk) and pushing it away from the brain tissue. (**c**) Reaching the anterior end of the AVM in the depth (arrow) where brain tissue can be seen (asterisk: AVM). (**d**) The posterior end (arrow) of the AVM (asterisk) is reached. (**e**) The surgical cavity after removal of the AVM

7.7.2 AVM of the Precentral Gyrus with Residual Hemorrhage

A comprehensive understanding of the 52 years old male patient's medical history unveiled a prolonged struggle with left-sided hemiplegia, a lasting consequence of an AVM rupture within the precentral gyrus a decade earlier. This AVM, showcased in Fig. 7.41, remained a constant threat of further hemorrhagic episodes, necessitating prompt and decisive intervention. Consequently, a critical decision was made to pursue surgical removal of the AVM in order to mitigate the possibility of subsequent bleeding events.

In preparation for this intricate procedure, an extensive craniotomy along the midline was meticulously performed. The surgical approach focused on tracing the aberrant and possibly pathological draining veins that visibly emerged on the surface and eventually led toward the AVM's core, or nidus. The preoperative imaging studies, particularly the magnetic resonance angiography (MRA), provided vital insights, suggesting that the arterial feeders likely emanated from the pericallosal arteries, indicating a deeper origin within the cerebral structure. Conversely, the anticipated drainage pathways

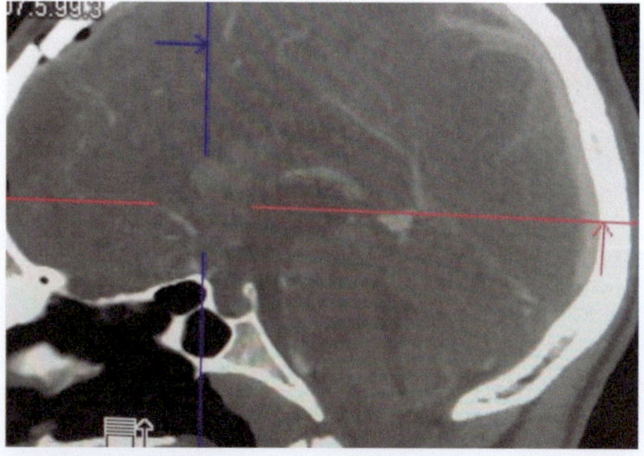

Fig. 7.40 Postoperative CTA after removal of the intraventricular AVM of Figs. 7.37, 7.38, and 7.39. The sagittal reconstructed CTA shows no signs of any AVM remnant. The hyperextended internal cerebral vein, which was seen preoperatively, is also not present

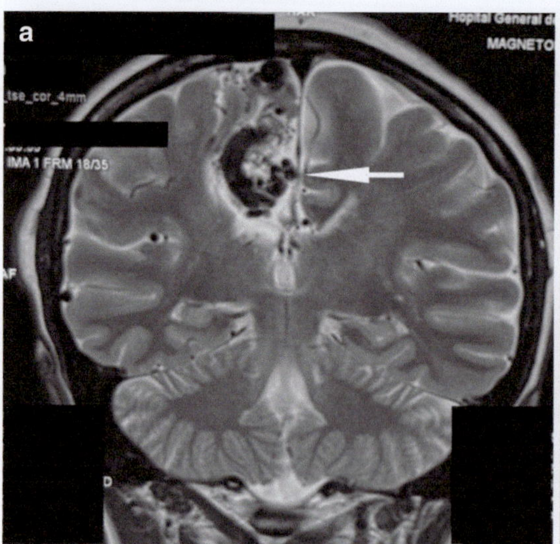
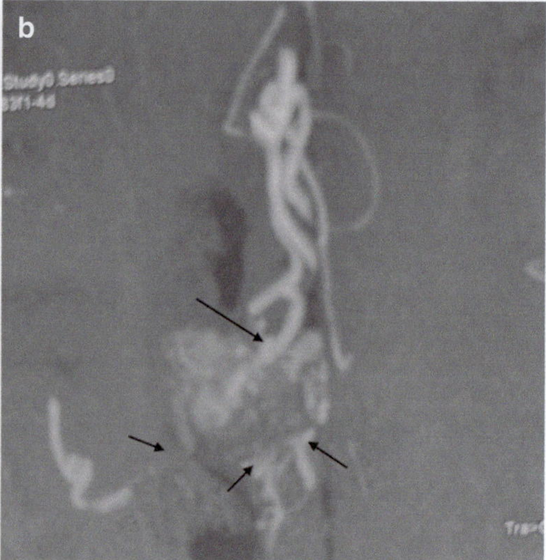
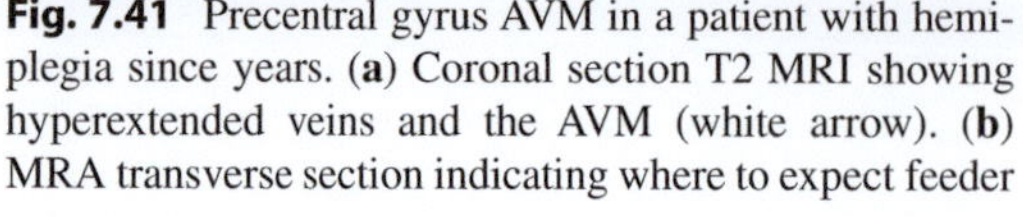

Fig. 7.41 Precentral gyrus AVM in a patient with hemiplegia since years. (**a**) Coronal section T2 MRI showing hyperextended veins and the AVM (white arrow). (**b**) MRA transverse section indicating where to expect feeder arteries (arrows). The feeding arteries are originating from the pericallosal artery mainly. More information cannot be gained by this MRA. DSA was not available

were expected to terminate at the superior sagittal sinus (SSS) and were more superficially located.

Guided by this intricate anatomical map, the surgical team meticulously navigated around the AVM's periphery. Employing a progressive approach from the surface toward the depths, they methodically dissected along the margins of the AVM. The objective was to progressively delve deeper, cautiously uncovering and systematically coagulating the principal feeder vessels as they emerged from within the depths of the AVM structure. As the surgical procedure advanced, these vital feeders, located prominently within the depths of the AVM, were identified and addressed.

Upon the strategic coagulation and management of these principal arterial feeders, the intricate removal of the entire AVM was achieved. This successful extraction, illustrating intricate surgical details, is showcased in the visual representations captured in Figs. 7.42 and 7.43. Through this precise and methodical surgical approach, the patient was afforded an opportunity for potential relief from the long-standing complications associated with the AVM, paving the way for a promising postoperative recovery and improved quality of life.

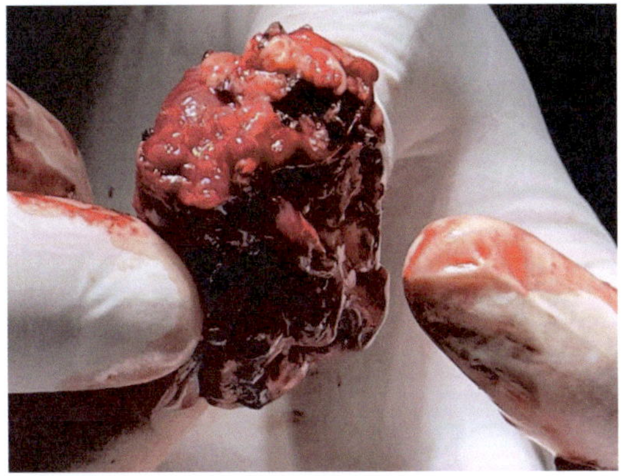

Fig. 7.42 Picture of the removed AVM. The surgical cavity was also free of any remaining tissue. Increasing the blood pressure to 150 mmHg systolic did not induce any bleeding into the cavity (not shown)

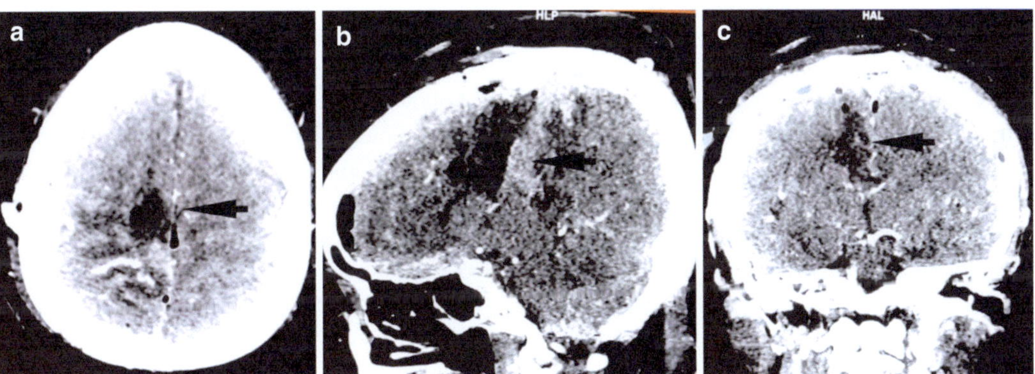

Fig. 7.43 Postoperative CTA of the patient from Fig. 7.41. (**a**) Transverse section of the CTA shows the cavity and no AVM (arrow). (**b**) The sagittal section of the CTA shows absent AVM (arrow) too. (**c**) The coronal reconstruction shows also no AVM remnants (arrow)

7.8 Spinal Intradural Arteriovenous Fistula

A young boy, merely 6 years old, presented with a progressive onset of paraparesis, gradually deteriorating to a point where he was rendered unable to walk independently. His neurological assessment indicated notable weakness in the lower limbs, graded at 2/5. The MRI examination revealed prominent dilation of intradural veins, specifically observed at the cervical levels C3 through C6, although the data depicting this finding is not available for reference.

In response to this concerning presentation, a surgical intervention was promptly organized. A laminectomy procedure targeting the cervical vertebrae C3 through C7 was performed as part of the initial approach. The entirety of the dura mater was meticulously opened along the midline, encompassing its full length, in a comprehensive effort to gain insight into the underlying pathology. Due to the unavailability of dynamic imaging techniques, the surgical team was compelled to rely on real-time observations of the vascular anatomy during the operation. This necessity led to an extensive and prolonged exposure of the dural region, essential for a thorough intraoperative assessment.

The preliminary diagnosis established during the surgical exploration pointed toward the presence of an arteriovenous spinal fistula. Notably, the right-sided radicular arteries at the C4 and C5 levels were identified as the likely feeders contributing to this pathologic condition. These arteries appeared to terminate within the dilated vein, indicative of the arteriovenous shunting, as illustrated in Fig. 7.44.

The absence of dynamic imaging techniques posed a considerable challenge during the procedure, necessitating a reliance on direct visual inspection to comprehend the intricacies of the arteriovenous malformation. Despite these limitations, the intraoperative findings provided crucial insights into the origin and dynamics of the spinal arteriovenous fistula, enabling the surgical team to initiate appropriate measures for further evaluation and management of this intricate vascular anomaly.

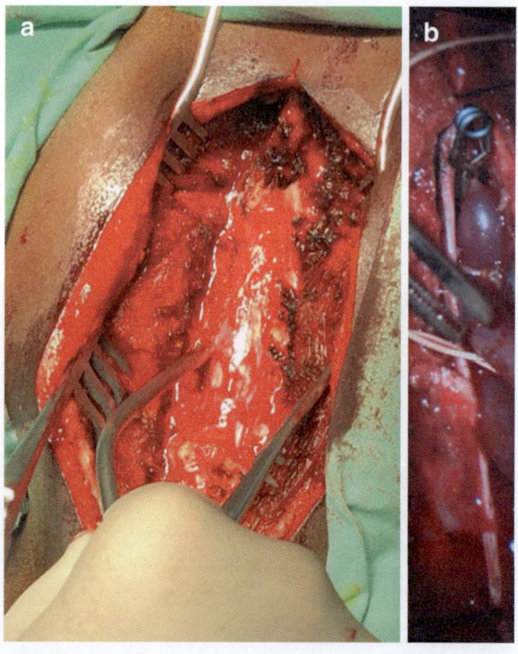

Fig. 7.44 A 6-year-old boy with paraplegia and an AVF of the cervical spine. Laminectomy C3-C7 revealing the dura. (**a**) After opening the dura over its midline from C3-C7, a distended vein compressing the spinal cord could be seen. (**b**) After coagulating the arteries, the vein was removed too in order to decompress the spinal cord

Following the identification of the affected vessels, a meticulous coagulation procedure was conducted, targeting both intra- and extradural arteries encircling the nerve roots. It's important to note that the integrity of these nerve structures was carefully preserved throughout the intervention. While addressing the vascular abnormality, the vein associated with the arteriovenous malformation exhibited thrombosis. However, due to its considerable size, a decision was made to surgically remove the thrombosed vein to prevent any potential complications, such as compression of the spinal cord or edema arising from inflammatory responses.

Immediatelly postsurgery, the patient's clinical condition did not exhibit any discernible improvement. The lower limb weakness and inability to walk persisted in the initial 3 months of follow-up. However, in the subsequent 6-month-postoperative assessment, a remarkable transformation was observed. Against our initial expectations, the patient displayed significant progress, demonstrating the ability to independently ambulate and walk. This noteworthy improvement in the clinical status, exceeding our initial prognostic expectations, aligns with findings documented in certain literature reports. These reports similarly indicate the potential for considerable recovery over the long term, often spanning several months, following surgical intervention for spinal arteriovenous fistulas (as depicted in Fig. 7.45).

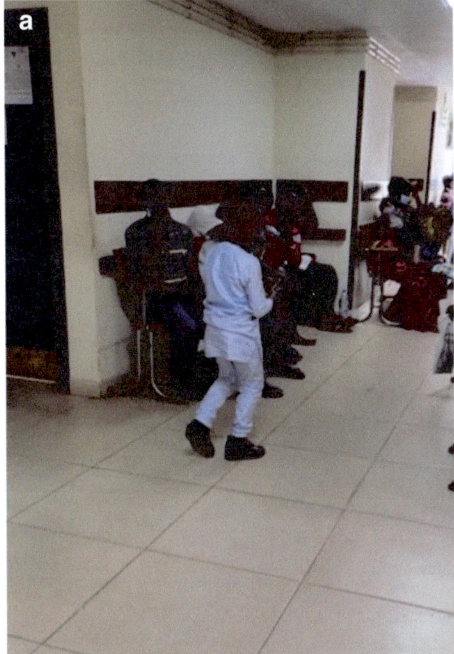
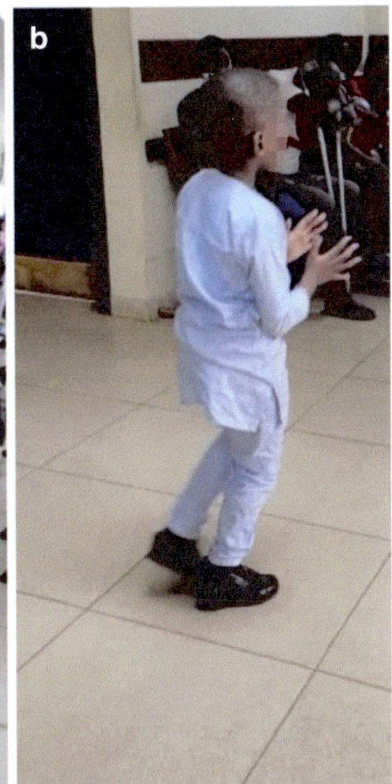

Fig. 7.45 (**a** and **b**) 6 months after removal of the cervical spinal AVF, the initially paraplegic young gentleman was able to walk again

Cultivate Trust in Your Senses: Journey Across Space and Time

8

During the surgical series conducted in Africa, as illustrated in the cases within this book, the assessment of intraoperative outcomes heavily relies on the direct examination of blood vessels and tactile feedback using the dissector. When dealing with an aneurysm, we employ a hands-on approach, relying on the sense of touch to detect any tension within the aneurysm, indicating potential incomplete occlusion and residual perfusion. If tension is sensed, we readjust the clip placement. Once confident in the clip's position, we cautiously introduce a syringe into the aneurysm. The absence of pulsating bleeding confirms successful occlusion. Should bleeding not occur, we open the aneurysm and carefully remove any thrombotic material. This manual and sensory-driven approach is crucial in ensuring the effectiveness of the surgical intervention.

Through this strategic method, we conduct a comprehensive assessment of the vessels surrounding the aneurysm to eliminate any potential risk of inadvertent arterial clip occlusion, which could result in compromised blood supply and subsequent tissue infarction. Before applying a clip to occlude an aneurysm, a detailed examination of the adjacent arteries is performed to detect any changes in their luminal structure following the application of the aneurysm clip.

Should the clip be situated too proximally to the artery of origin, inducing constriction in the neighboring vessels, a meticulous evaluation of the arteries' lumens is conducted. The clip is carefully reopened, allowing for a visual assessment of the arterial filling. If there's a noticeable discrepancy suggesting compromised blood flow, the clip is readjusted, repositioned 1–2 mm away from the artery, ensuring it aligns precisely with the aneurysm neck. This maneuver allows for a controlled remnant of the aneurysm while maintaining adequate blood flow through the adjacent arteries, reducing the risk of ischemic complications.

If intraoperative angiography like indocyanine green video-angiography or micro-Doppler was available, the assessment of aneurysm perfusion or identification of adjacent vessel stenoses would be significantly more accessible and reliable. This advanced technology would also decrease the likelihood of leaving behind a small residual aneurysm. A comprehensive study highlighting the strengths and limitations of each intraoperative method, such as digital subtraction angiography (DSA), indocyanine green (ICG), and micro-Doppler, exists in the literature [42]. Typically, developed nations with specialized neurovascular centers employ a combination of ICG and micro-Doppler for enhanced intraoperative monitoring [42].

In a notable case conducted in Germany, Fig. 8.1 portrays the treatment of a giant non-ruptured aneurysm employing ICG angiography for intraoperative control of arterial perfusion. Furthermore,

Fig. 8.1 Surgery of a giant MCA aneurysm in Germany. (**a**) The calcified giant aneurysm in the Sylvan fissure is identified together with the aneurysm neck. (**b**) A clip is applied in the aneurysm neck. (**c**) The aneurysm is opened, and the thrombus is removed. Inspection into the aneurysm sack allows to define where the M2 arteries are leaving the aneurysm. Part of the aneurysm wall is used to allow perfusion of the adjacent arteries. Only through opening the aneurysm, we can inspect the exact clip placement. (**d**) Intraoperative inspection of the clip position and the relation of the clip to the M2 artery. (**e**) Intraoperative ICG video-angiography shows excellent perfusion of both M2 arteries. (**f**) Postoperative CTA reconstruction, showing no aneurysm and the presence of M2 arteries

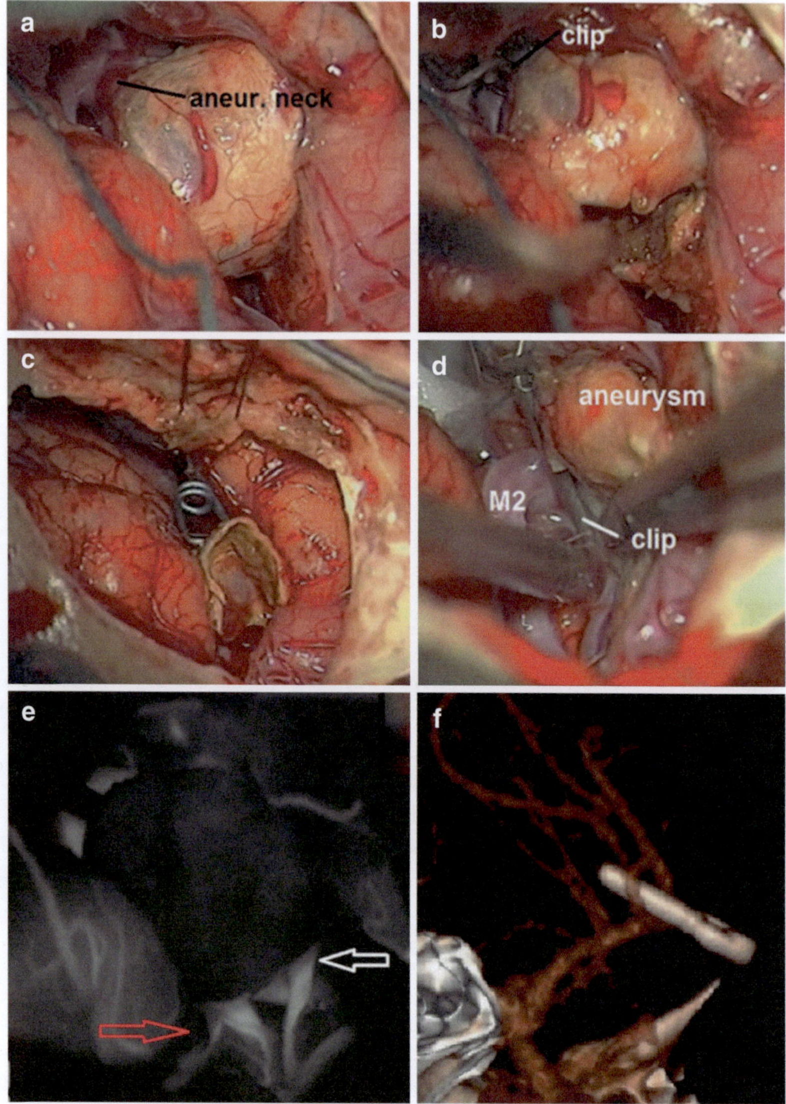

Fig. 8.2 depicts the clipping of a giant ruptured aneurysm utilizing ICG as a video-angiography method for precise intraoperative monitoring.

The dilemma persists within bypass surgeries in low-income countries, where the absence of sophisticated technology necessitates reliance on sensory evaluation. Verification of bypass functionality primarily involves assessing the saphenous vein postimplantation. Pulsation and adequate filling are indicative of an intact bypass, allowing surgeons to ascertain its viability. The absence of pulsation signals a potential issue with the bypass. In such instances, a comprehensive examination of the bypass is conducted, encompassing palpation along its entire length. When identification of a thrombus occurs and attempts at vessel massage fail to resolve the obstruction, surgical intervention involves incising the affected vessel to remove the thrombus. Subsequently, the incision is meticulously repaired using 7-0 stitches to restore vessel integrity.

Moreover, an additional challenge frequently encountered is the suboptimal quality of the imaging scans obtained from patients admitted from other hospitals. These images, often in the

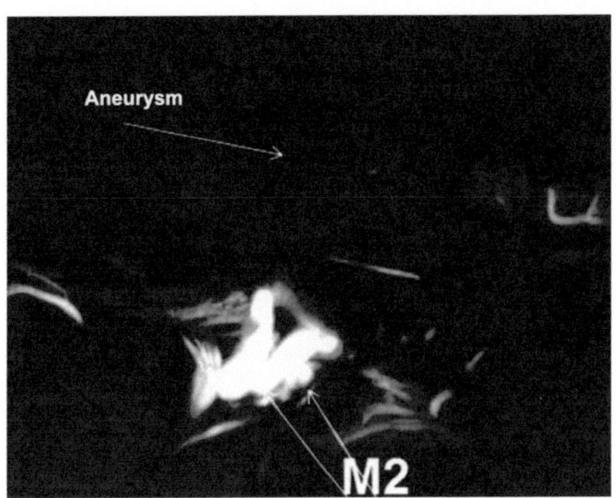

Fig. 8.2 Intraoperative ICG video-angiography in Germany. A giant MCA aneurysm is clipped, and ICG video-angiography is performed to reassure perfusion of the M2 coming out of the giant aneurysm, which is clip reconstructed

form of printed MRI or CTA scans, may possess thick slices and inadequate resolution. Despite the potential benefits of obtaining clearer, higher-resolution images through repeat examinations at the reference hospital, some patients may decline this option, possibly due to various factors, including financial constraints or reluctance to undergo further tests. This predicament poses a challenge for surgical planning, as clearer imaging is crucial for precise preoperative evaluation and strategizing.

The localization of an aneurysm within the cerebral vasculature is a crucial aspect in its surgical management. Identification of its point of origin from a specific vessel guides our approach during the surgical procedure. Achieving a comprehensive understanding of the precise anatomy, particularly the configuration of the aneurysm neck and its relationship with adjacent vessels, demands meticulous dissection during the operation.

However, challenges often arise, especially with the imaging quality of CT angiography (CTA) in cases involving aneurysms around the AcomA (anterior communicating artery) complex. The ambiguity may arise regarding whether the aneurysm originates from the left A1-A2 or the right, presenting difficulty in determining the precise origin. Sometimes, the surgical approach

is initiated from the side where the dome of the aneurysm is encountered rather than the neck. Nevertheless, the surgical team systematically progresses from the dome toward the neck, eventually identifying and occluding the neck with a clip. Surgeons, when encountering such scenarios, need to approach the aneurysm with heightened awareness that what they initially visualize could potentially be the ruptured dome not the actual neck. In the unfortunate event of re-rupture, dissection needs to focus around the aneurysm, tracing from the dome to accurately locate and address the neck.

Once the intricate anatomy is meticulously clarified, the selection of the appropriate clip becomes imperative. Surgeons are tasked with making judicious decisions, aiming to use as few clips as possible while ensuring complete and effective aneurysm occlusion. This strategy involves careful consideration of the ideal clip placement to achieve optimal occlusion and minimize the risks associated with multiple clips and their potential impact on adjacent vessels.

Avoiding the use of multiple clips during clip occlusion is crucial due to potential limitations in the number of clips available, especially during surgical missions in low-resource settings. Utilizing numerous clips might exhaust the clip inventory, potentially preventing further clipping procedures during the expert surgeon's tenure. Therefore, it becomes the responsibility of the expert surgeon to assess the upcoming cases they will handle during their stay and anticipate the quantity and types of clips required to ensure the availability of adequate resources.

Effective planning and preparation are essential aspects of the surgeon's role, necessitating them to forecast the necessary clip types and quantities required for each surgical procedure. This proactive approach aims to prevent any instances where a shortage of clips impedes the completion of critical surgeries. To facilitate this planning process, innovative technologies such as 3D printing can be highly beneficial. Creating 3D-printed models of aneurysms based on CTA data can aid surgeons in preoperative planning and strategizing the specific clips needed for each case.

In the context of surgical missions in Africa, there's an opportunity to leverage modern communication and printing technologies. CTAs of patients in Africa could be transmitted to the expert surgeon, who, using a 3D printer at their home institution, could replicate the aneurysm models. By doing so, the expert surgeon can meticulously plan and simulate the surgeries that will be performed in developing countries, ensuring precise preparation and adequate resource allocation before undertaking the actual procedures. This innovative approach enhances surgical preparedness and minimizes the risk of clip shortages during critical interventions in underserved regions.

While I deeply appreciate the value of technical advancements, I also firmly believe in the power of human intuition and the ability to rely on one's senses, especially in situations where technological aids may falter or prove insufficient. There exists a crucial juncture where technology reaches its limitations, and this is where human ingenuity and improvisation come into play. The capability to improvise is a vital human skill that demands constant refinement and honing.

Embracing improvisation doesn't imply disregarding technical tools but rather understanding their limitations and being prepared for situations where they might fall short. It's a challenge to visualize the intricate anatomy of an aneurysm, observe it during surgery, and assess how closely the reality aligns with our preoperative mental plans. Recognizing the disparities between our preconceptions and the actual scenario is crucial; it's through these insights that we learn and evolve for future procedures.

In our approach, we don't rely on preoperative 3D printing to simulate aneurysm anatomy before our on-site fellowship. Instead, we ensure a comprehensive collection of clips, mitigating any risk of clip shortages during our tenure. For instance, fenestrated straight and 90° angulated clips serve as versatile alternatives for securing aneurysms on the posterior wall of arteries. Even if originally intended for specific purposes, these clips can adapt to other needs if standard clips are unavailable. Therefore, we lean toward prioritizing these versatile clips, constituting about 75% of our inventory, to preempt any clip shortage contingencies. This strategy allows us to maintain a higher level of readiness during surgeries in resource-limited settings.

In essence, it's the amalgamation of technological assistance and human adaptability that enables us to navigate the challenges of neurosurgery in varied circumstances, aiming for optimal patient care and successful surgical outcomes.

9.1 Patients After Aneurysm Surgery

After the closure of the surgical incision, the external ventricular drain (EVD) was removed in the operating room, and the patients were successfully extubated. It's important to note that the aneurysms had ruptured weeks to months before the surgery, and the patients were fully conscious before the procedure commenced. Postsurgery, all patients were promptly shifted to the intensive care unit (ICU) for close monitoring and received nimodipine at a dosage of 60 mg three times a day. This medication was administered empirically to prevent potential vasospasms resulting from any manipulation of the vessels during surgery (no evidence based)

The patients' blood pressure was meticulously regulated to maintain normotensive levels, with a maximum systolic pressure of 140 mmHg. Additionally, their fluid intake was carefully controlled, limited to 2 L within a 24-h period. The subsequent day following surgery, each patient underwent a postsurgical CTA (computed tomography angiography) or CCT (computed tomography scan). After a 48-h postoperative period, they were transferred from the ICU to the regular ward for further care, where they remained under observation for an additional 5–7 days.

If any postoperative neurological deterioration was observed in the patients, an immediate computed tomography (CCT) and computed tomog-raphy angiography (CTA) were conducted. These diagnostic tests were essential to rule out hydrocephalus or infarctions. If these conditions were excluded and vasospasm was suspected, the patients were prescribed a full dose of nimodipine at 60 mg, administered orally six times a day for the subsequent 14 days. Additionally, a moderate increase in blood pressure was allowed, with the systolic pressure raised to a maximum of 160 mmHg.

In cases where symptoms persisted despite this regimen, the systolic blood pressure was further increased to a maximum of 200 mmHg. However, it's important to note that intra-arterial administration of nimodipine via angiography or balloon dilatation was not a viable option due to the unavailability of angio-catheterization.

Throughout the fellowship program, the expert and fellows maintained a close monitoring schedule, visiting patients twice daily in the ICU and once daily in the regular ward. Routine blood tests were conducted daily, and all patients received antibiotic treatment until the day of discharge to ensure optimal recovery and prevent infections.

9.2 Patients After AVM Surgery

Following the removal of arteriovenous malformations (AVMs), it was the preferred protocol to keep patients in the intensive care unit (ICU)

A. K. Petridis, H. Maslehaty, *Vascular Neurosurgery in Environments with Limited Resources*, https://doi.org/10.1007/978-3-031-59675-9_9

without intubation for a period of 4–6 days. Blood pressure management was a critical aspect of postoperative care, ensuring that blood pressure remained below 130 mmHg for the initial 3 days. This cautious approach aimed to prevent potential risks associated with hyperperfusion injury and the occurrence of intracerebral bleeding. The emphasis on maintaining optimal blood pressure levels was crucial in safeguarding against postoperative complications and ensuring a smoother recovery process.

9.3   Patients After Bypass Surgery

The bypass surgeries (STA-MCA; carotid—saphenous vein—MCA) performed in Cameroon and Tanzania were groundbreaking achievements in the region, marking the first instances of such procedures in these countries, as far as our information extended. However, postsurgical protocols for treating these patients were not standardized. Ensuring the patency of the bypasses became a paramount concern.

To address this, a meticulous regimen was established. Immediately after surgery, patients were commenced on aspirin 100 mg. Additionally, a weight-adjusted heparin treatment regimen was initiated on the subsequent day. Notably, patients were not preloaded with heparin before the surgery due to the risk of potential complications, specifically the danger of compressing the donor vessel caused by local hematomas, which was observed in one of our two high-flow bypass patients.

The critical need to maintain bypass patency led to a delicate balance between anticoagulation therapy and avoiding potential risks, shaping the postoperative care strategy for these pioneering procedures in the region.

In our complicative case where the bypass was occluded by a subcutaneous hematoma, we proceeded as follows:

Following the completion of the bypass procedure, the patient was promptly transferred to the intensive care unit (ICU) with explicit instructions for rigorous neurological evaluations to be conducted every 20 min during the initial 4 h postsurgery, transitioning to hourly evaluations thereafter.

During the initial 2-h postoperative period, the patient demonstrated an optimal neurological status, exhibiting responsiveness to commands and exhibiting full mobility in all four extremities without any signs of weakness. However, a concerning development emerged after this period, marked by the onset of weakness on the contralateral side.

Further examination revealed the presence of a cranial subcutaneous hematoma, exerting pressure on the bypass. Swift action was taken to alleviate this complication by promptly removing the hematoma, consequently restoring the integrity and functionality of the bypass.

Emphasizing the critical nature of ICU care, it's vital to underscore that meticulous and continuous patient examination and observation represent indispensable aspects of postoperative management, not only in low-income countries but universally across all medical settings worldwide. This vigilant monitoring ensures early detection and prompt intervention in response to emergent complications, contributing significantly to enhanced patient outcomes and recovery.

In order to establish a comprehensive training program and effectively evaluate its outcomes and advancements, maintaining a stance of self-criticism and honesty remains our primary ally. Our observation of patient cases spans from the inception of surgery to an ongoing timeline, which extends for a minimum of 5 years. All patients are subjected to microsurgical interventions, thereby obviating the necessity for regular DSA (digital subtraction angiography) or MRA (magnetic resonance angiography) follow-up examinations, as they haven't undergone any endovascular treatments. CTA is satisfying enough as a follow-up control, since it is readily available and inexpensive.

Postsurgical follow-ups are meticulously conducted at designated intervals: at 3 months, 6 months, 1 year, and subsequently every 2 years thereafter. These follow-ups entail CTA (computed tomography angiography) examinations aimed at detecting any residual perfusion anomalies or potential emergence of new aneurysms in other vessels.

This approach not only serves to monitor the progress and recuperation of the treated patients but also aids in identifying any latent risks or unforeseen developments, thus allowing for proactive intervention and comprehensive patient care.

In a particular study of Vourla et al., the risk of developing de novo aneurysms was reported at 7.6%, and these newly formed aneurysms surfaced over an average duration of 7.9 years. This emphasizes the critical importance of extended, ongoing monitoring of individuals diagnosed with intracranial aneurysms. Notably, in their series, a majority of the newly formed aneurysms emerged after a follow-up period exceeding 5 years [43]. This observation highlights the necessity for prolonged surveillance and vigilance in managing patients with a history of intracranial aneurysms, enabling early detection and intervention to mitigate potential risks.

To effectively identify any new aneurysms, the follow-up time interval should span at least 7 years. Throughout this follow-up period, our assessment encompasses various crucial aspects such as the Glasgow Outcome Scale (GOS) evaluation, monitoring discomfort levels, examining aesthetic outcomes, scrutinizing motor and cognitive functions, and assessing the patients' ability to return to work. However, it's important to note that a considerable number of patients do not actively participate in these follow-up examinations. This low participation rate is often attributed to significant factors such as long distances to the hospital, which incur additional costs for transportation, along with expenses associated with the required CTA imaging.

To bridge this gap, our next step involves reaching out to these patients via telephone, allowing us to communicate with them and gain insights into their well-being. Many patients, despite being in good health, express a reluctance to physically visit the hospital for these follow-up examinations. Nevertheless, we make concerted efforts to emphasize the significance of these check-ups and endeavor to educate patients about the critical importance in ensuring continued health and early detection of any potential issues.

Continuous Education and Remote Case Deliberations 11

Certainly, supporting and guiding local neurosurgeons in a specialized field necessitates more than just performing surgeries. It encompasses various facets of education and mentorship. Addressing inquiries that arise, supervising patient wound management, assessing follow-up CTAs, and imparting knowledge about updated guidelines and recent breakthroughs in the literature are fundamental aspects. Equally vital is conducting a thorough analysis of the expert's surgical procedures, both complex and routine cases conducted in their native country, alongside evaluations of surgeries performed by the trainees in the expert's absence. This comprehensive approach forms an integral part of any effective educational program in this domain.

These educational webinars occur on a monthly basis, offering a regular platform for learning and discussion. Immediate solutions to any urgent queries are addressed through prompt online communication within hours or a few days at most.

The expert neurosurgeon remains informed about postoperative complications, follow-up assessments, and new cases, remaining available to provide guidance and advice as needed. In situations where the expert perceives a case as too challenging for the newly trained vascular surgeons, they make arrangements to personally visit the hospital and perform the surgery.

The webinars organized for the fellows and residents cover a wide array of topics, including surgical approaches, techniques in vascular surgery, management of subarachnoid hemorrhages, comparative analysis of microsurgery and endovascular procedures, considerations of cost-effectiveness, intensive care unit (ICU) treatment for subarachnoid hemorrhage, bypass surgery techniques, and indications, among other key subjects.

To effectively train fellows, they must engage in the entire thought process of their mentor. It's not only about replicating techniques but also comprehending the rationale behind their mentor's thinking and learning to adopt a similar mindset. Much like in the learning process of artificial intelligence (AI), fellows need to reevaluate procedures, adapt them, and seek ways to enhance them. A competent fellow isn't just someone who imitates; they grasp the underlying principles and logic. A proficient educator elucidates to the fellows not just what is done, but why a specific approach is chosen over others.

An expert should strive to articulate their thoughts clearly, allowing the team to comprehend and actively engage in the decision-making behind each surgical maneuver. Similar to the learning patterns observed in young children, the learning process remains universal and consistent even in adulthood. Learning inherently prompts a fundamental question: "… but why?" This universal inquiry is at the heart of the learning process.

A. K. Petridis, H. Maslehaty, *Vascular Neurosurgery in Environments with Limited Resources*,
https://doi.org/10.1007/978-3-031-59675-9_11

If we extrapolate the demographic data from the western world to the African population, the anticipated incidence of aSAH (aneurysmal subarachnoid hemorrhage) should fall within the range of 2–22 cases per 100,000 patients per year, as cited in ref. [3] of the paper. Considering the population of the Yaounde area, which stands at approximately 2.7 million, the projected incidence of aSAH would theoretically range between 55 and 608 cases annually. Even if we account for a mortality rate of 25% for immediate deaths following aSAH, the estimated incidence would still be around 41–456 cases per year.

In contrast, the observed incidence rate in Yaounde, particularly in the reference hospital specializing in cerebrovascular pathologies, is only 25 cases per year. This significantly lower figure implies that individuals experiencing SAH might not be receiving appropriate treatment or are potentially overlooked within the healthcare system, resulting in underdiagnosis and undertreatment of aSAH cases.

For the population of Cameroon, which stands at 27.2 million, the anticipated number of individuals affected by aneurysms based on global incidence rates would approximate around 1.28 million cases. This substantial number highlights a pressing need for specialized centers of excellence dedicated to the accurate diagnosis and management of aneurysms within the country.

In addressing this growing demand for neurosurgical care, the experience and expertise of local surgeons in Africa are poised to surpass that of their counterparts in the Western world. As African neurosurgeons encounter a progressively higher volume of cases, their confidence and proficiency in handling complex procedures, such as aneurysm treatments, are expected to increase significantly. This growth in expertise not only benefits the local healthcare system but also contributes to elevating the standard of neurosurgical care on a global scale.

In order to provide comprehensive care for all patients affected by aSAH in developing countries, there is a critical need for widespread education within the population. Initially, raising awareness among the populace is crucial, starting with informing them about the establishment of a dedicated center of excellence within their own country. Introducing this center to the public becomes paramount.

Various communication channels, such as interviews, newspaper articles, and media reports, should be utilized to disseminate information regarding cerebrovascular diseases and their treatment modalities. These informative sessions will serve to educate the population about the prevalence, symptoms, risk factors, and available management options for cerebrovascular pathologies like aSAH. By enhancing public awareness, individuals can recognize symptoms early,

A. K. Petridis, H. Maslehaty, *Vascular Neurosurgery in Environments with Limited Resources*,
https://doi.org/10.1007/978-3-031-59675-9_12

seek timely medical attention, and gain trust in local healthcare resources for effective treatment and management.

We initiated a comprehensive public education campaign through TV and newspaper interviews (Fig. 12.1). This proactive approach ensured that information about our efforts and achievements in treating cerebrovascular conditions reached a wider audience. Moreover, we periodically shared the outcomes from nearly 50% of the treated cases with the local newspapers (Fig. 12.2). This approach wasn't just about highlighting our successes; it was crucial in fostering trust within the community and dispelling misconceptions about hospitals being solely a place for dire circumstances rather than a place to restore health.

By disseminating information about successful treatment outcomes, we aimed to shift the perception of hospitals from sites of despair to institutions dedicated to restoring health and well-being. It was imperative for us to instill confidence in the local population, assuring them that seeking medical help was not a futile endeavor but rather a step toward recovery and improved health.

Upon the conclusion of the fellowship in Cameroon, a formal ceremony was held to introduce the two new vascular neurosurgeons, along with the center and the surgical outcomes achieved during the program, to the wider public. This was accomplished through coverage by major national and private TV stations as well as prominent newspapers. This ceremony served as an important means to further strengthen the bond between the medical community and the public, building a sense of solidarity and trust in local healthcare initiatives.

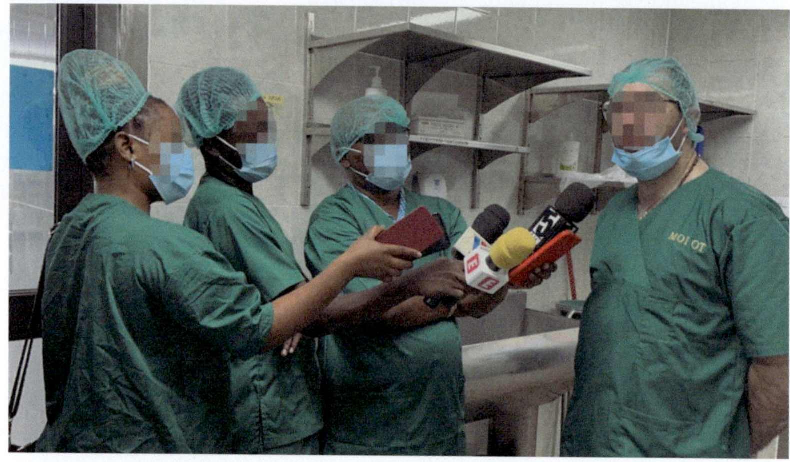

Fig. 12.1 Educating the public through TV interviews about vascular neurosurgical pathologies and the fellowship program in general

Fig. 12.2 Title page of the newspaper Echo Sante (with permission to publish here) stating the interim results of the fellowship. The title states that 25 patient (maladies cardio et neuro-vasculaire = cardio and neurovascular diseases as a category) had been operated in the General Hospital in Yaounde, together with a picture of Athanasios Petridis and his two fellows. In the article, the fellowship program is introduced to the public

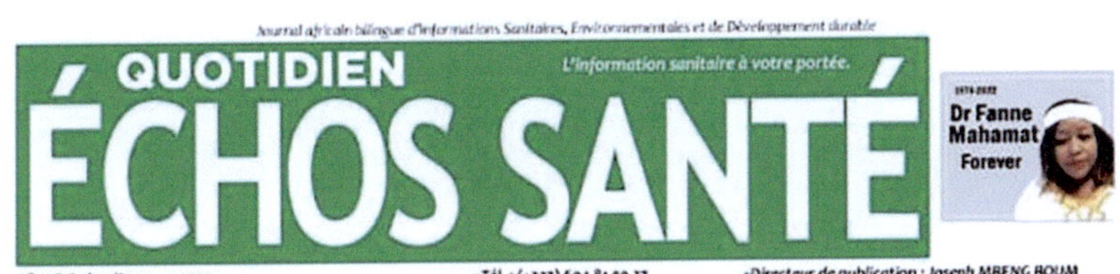

Journal africain bilingue d'Informations Sanitaires, Environnementales et de Développement durable

QUOTIDIEN

ÉCHOS SANTÉ

L'information sanitaire à votre portée.

•N° 458 du lundi 21 mars 2022   •Tél. : (+237) 694 81 99 37   •Directeur de publication : Joseph MBENG BOUM

Maladies cardio et neuro-vasculaires

25 patients opérés à l'Hôpital Général de Yaoundé

Une campagne d'opérations des patients souffrant des pathologies de neurochirurgies vasculaires au Cameroun a été organisée par le Directeur Général, de l'Hôpital Général de Yaoundé, le Pr Vincent de Paul Djientcheu, Neurochirurgien et son collègue Allemand, le Pr. Petridis Athanasios, Spécialiste en neurochirurgie vasculaire. Pendant deux semaines, 25 malades ont été opérés avec succès dans cette formation sanitaire de référence de la ville de Yaoundé. Pages 6-7

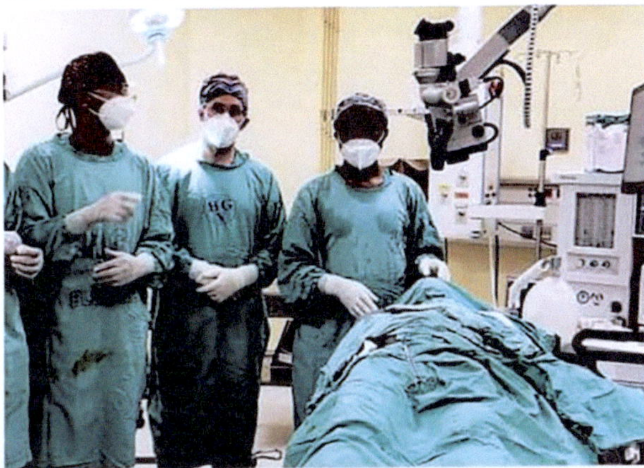

Hôpital militaire de région N° 2 de Douala

Une campagne de chirurgie du Noma lancée

Une opération d'intervention chirurgicale des malformations du visage, dirigée par l'association du Noma en collaboration avec le ministère de la Défense, l'Ordre National des Médecins du Cameroun et la fondation Foe, se tient depuis lundi 14 mars 2022 à la garnison de Douala. Page 5

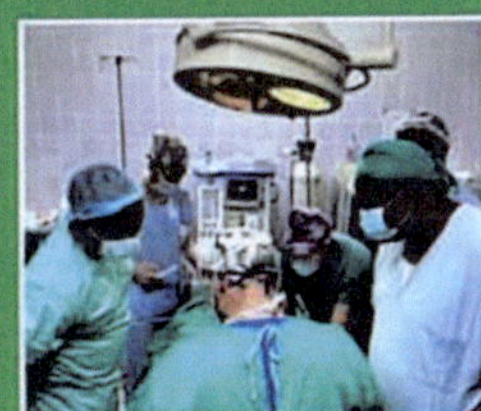

Sante maternelle et néonatale

Les infirmiers accoucheurs remettent à jour leurs connaissances à Garoua

Depuis une semaine, ils prennent part à un séminaire de formation en soins obstétricaux et néonataux d'urgence, animé par l'Association des compétences pour une vie meilleure (ASCOVIME) et l'ONG Gynécologie Sans Frontières. Objectif, diminuer le taux de mortalité de la mère et de l'enfant dans le septentrion du Cameroun, taux jusqu'ici élevé. Page 10

w w w . e c h o s a n t e . i n f o

13.1 Cameroon

After the successful completion of the inaugural "reverse" or "on-site" fellowship in Cameroon, the two newly trained vascular neurosurgeons demonstrated their proficiency by independently performing microsurgical clipping procedures for ruptured ICA and pcomA aneurysms, without direct supervision. Although the expert was present during the surgeries, he did not intervene or actively participate. Despite this, the duration of microscope use was only 30 min, demonstrating the surgeons' efficiency. Notably, the aneurysms were completely occluded, and the procedures transpired without any intraoperative complications. Importantly, there were no disturbances in the perfusion of neighboring vessels, and post-surgery, the patients promptly regained consciousness without any neurological deficits.

This milestone in training signifies the onset of a new era in neurovascular care in Cameroon. Patients who were previously not receiving treatment for aSAH will hopefully now seek admission to the center, fostering a ray of hope for many lives to be saved in the future. This pivotal achievement not only ensures the immediate care of those afflicted but also signifies the establishment of a foundation for improved neurovascular health care in the region, offering prospects for enhanced treatment, better outcomes, and, ultimately, a positive impact on the community's well-being.

The surgeries conducted under the supervision of the expert exhibited comparable morbidity and mortality rates to those observed in developing countries. The cumulative morbidity rate stood at 10.5%, with a long-term functional morbidity rate of 5.2%. There were no intraoperative mortalities recorded, while the 30-day mortality rate remained at 2.7%. The average duration of the operation, from incision to closure, spanned approximately 125 min (ranging between 60 and 220 min), taking into consideration the predominant use of the Gigly saw for craniotomies. Microscope utilization varied from 12 to 80 min, contingent on the pace of dissection by the fellows during the surgical procedures.

In assessing the performance of the fellows following the completion of their vascular neurosurgery fellowship, their outcomes were compared against their surgical results pre-fellowship. Prior to undertaking the fellowship, 13 patients underwent aneurysm surgeries without subarachnoid hemorrhage (SAH), with an average operating time of 5 h and 30 min. During this period, there were two reported deaths within the initial 30-day postoperative phase, along with two cases of significant postsurgical morbidity. Unfortunately, detailed specifics regarding the nature of the morbidity and mortality, as well as follow-up data, were not available.

Subsequent to the completion of the vascular fellowship program, the two local trainees independently performed 15 surgeries for non-ruptured aneurysms. Encouragingly, these surgeries yielded no surgical complications or fatalities. Notably, the operating time for these cases was reduced to an average of 4 h and 15 min.

13.2 Tanzania

The data collected from Tanzania revealed some variance in outcomes. Remarkably, six out of eight patients (75%) demonstrated excellent surgical outcomes, experiencing no complications or postoperative morbidity. Unfortunately, the remaining two patients succumbed to adverse events during an extended ICU stay. These events were attributed to perfusion deficits, resulting in cerebral infarctions. Consequently, the mortality rate within the initial 30 days postsurgery reached an unexpectedly high 25%.

Efforts to address these challenges involve conducting morbidity and mortality conferences and leveraging the dedication of the fellows. These initiatives are aimed at instigating change and improvement in the observed rates, with the primary goal of enhancing patient outcomes.

13.3 Summary

Assuming responsibility for training an entire new generation of vascular neurosurgeons in low-income regions like Central Africa is not just an honor but also the realization of a long-awaited dream. Acting as a common supervisor for these new vascular surgeons, who initially acquired their techniques from us, prompts immense interest in witnessing and guiding their professional development. Their evolving skill set, shaped by their caseload and expanding experience, is of profound significance to us as it also drives our own growth and evolution in this field.

If these newly trained neurosurgeons advance and refine the techniques they've learned from their mentors, while still involving their teachers in their modifications, it signifies a continuous cycle of improvement. As experts in the field, we become an integral part of an evolutionary process, enhancing ourselves through the experiences and innovations of our students. The narrative of vascular neurosurgery in Africa will progress with the guidance of Western experts, imparting their skills to enthusiastic and gifted young neurosurgeons. Being present at the inception of this transformative history and playing a pivotal role in it is profound, profoundly touching, and will fundamentally alter the perspectives on surgical approaches for both the mentor and the learner, forever shaping their surgical philosophies.

When the teaching process commences and you convey your insights to your pupils, it initiates a deeper reflection within yourself. It compels you to articulate to your own mind the rationale behind each surgical step. You actively engage with your own technique, allowing those subconscious processes to emerge into your conscious awareness. Teaching isn't merely instructing others; it's an act of instructing yourself. By articulating and elucidating the surgical procedures to your students, you're essentially clarifying, reflecting, and refining your own understanding. This interactive process encourages introspection, enabling you to reconsider certain steps, rectify any errors, discover more effective approaches, and, consequently, enhance your own proficiency.

Upon completion of the fellowships across numerous countries in central Africa, a new cohort of vascular neurosurgeons will emerge, equipped to confront ruptured aneurysms with a blend of confidence, reverence, and a profound understanding of managing intraoperative and postsurgical complications. Enhancing the healthcare infrastructure in these nations not only elevates the well-being of their citizens but also contributes to the enhancement of life quality in the western world. By empowering African countries with a robust health system, individuals will gradually repose trust in their local healthcare resources, potentially diminishing the desire to seek opportunities in more developed but distant countries. This transformation can foster a sense of hope within the local populace, reducing the yearning to migrate to what might have been perceived as a "more promising" world elsewhere.

To address the issue of illegal migration and the tragic loss of lives in search of a better life, I firmly believe that enhancing the quality of life within the countries people are fleeing from is paramount. A fundamental aspect of this improvement lies in bolstering the healthcare system. Rather than channeling substantial resources into fortifying borders to insulate a perceived "civilized" world, redirecting these investments toward enhancing the infrastructure of nations from which people are migrating would be a far more beneficial approach. It's essential to clarify that this viewpoint is personal (AKP) and not intended as a political stance.

As healthcare professionals working and closely observing life in low-income countries, we can form opinions and advocate for change without necessarily creating a political manifesto. The experience of working in these regions has been transformative for me personally, one that I wouldn't trade for anything and which has shaped my perspective in profound ways.

Figures 13.1 and 13.2 show the daily work in Cameroon and Tanzania as well as the hospital facility and the out-of-hospital environment, and Fig. 13.3 shows the lack of power after a full week or weeks of cerebrovascular surgeries in central Africa.

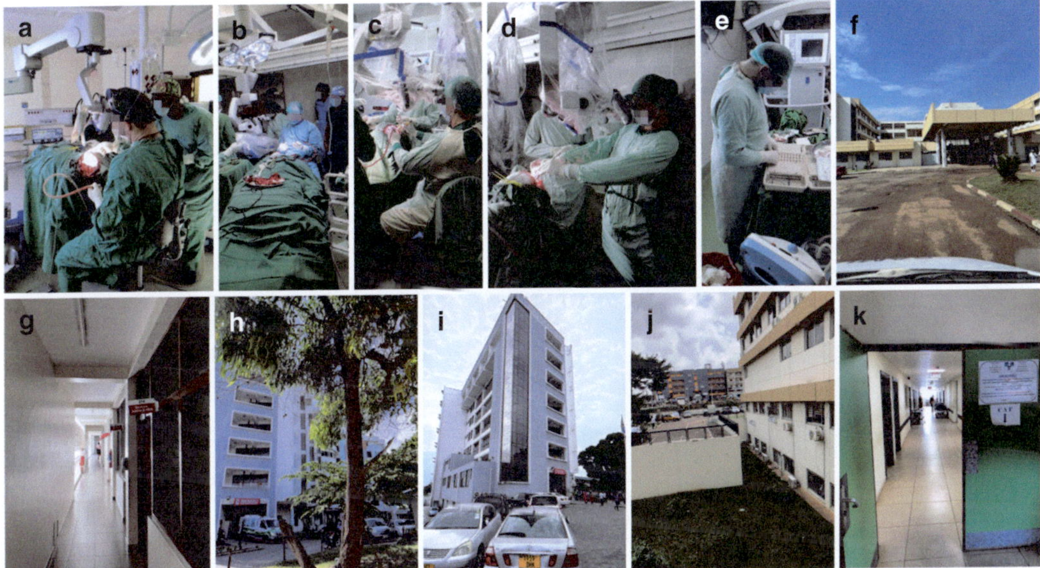

Fig. 13.1 Daily routine in Africa. These are some images insight the operating rooms and the facilities we are working at. (**a–d**) Surgical performance. Sitting or standing (**d**). (**e**) Inspecting the micro-instruments and preselecting clips, as well as checking the clip appliers and functionality of the micro-instruments. You can take nothing for granted, since the expert is the one who knows how instruments should perform. (**f**) Entrance of the Yaounde General Hospital, Cameroon. (**g**) Offices in MUHAS, Tanzania. (**h and i**) The department of orthopedics and neurosurgery in MUHAS, Tanzania. (**j and k**) Yaounde General Hospital, Cameroon

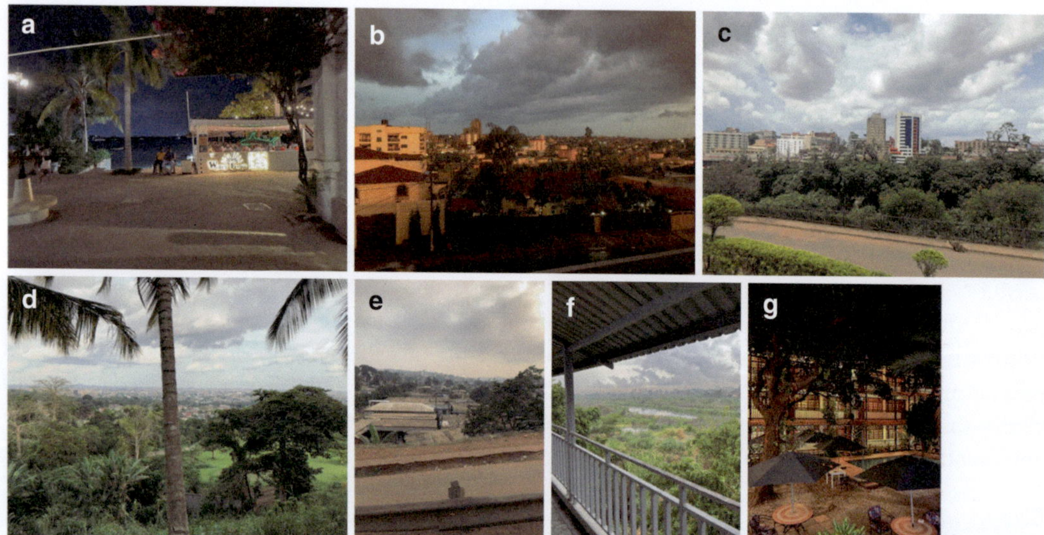

Fig. 13.2 A life outside the hospital. (**a**) Seaside in Dar Es Salam, Tanzania, with cocktail bars and fish restaurants. (**b**) View outside the hotel in Yaounde, Cameroon. (**c**) Yaounde seen from a city park. (**d**) Up the hill in Yaounde. (**e**) View from the hospital to the city of Yaounde. (**f**) View from MUHAS to a river close to the hospital. (**g**) The accommodation in Tanzania

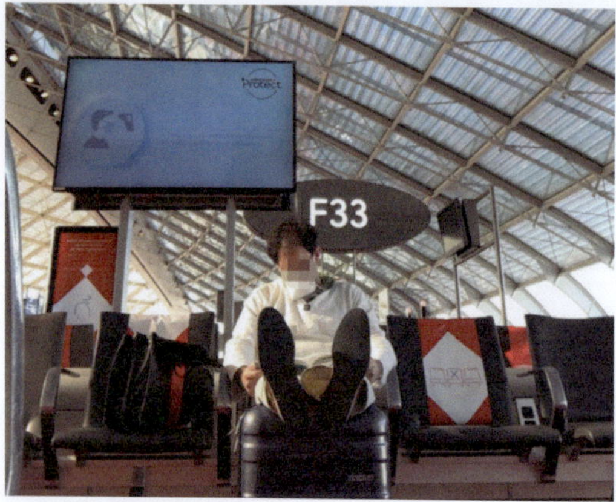

Fig. 13.3 After 2 weeks of surgeries in Africa. Exhaustion and satisfaction

References

1. Kamiguchi H, Shiobara R, Toya S. Accidentally detected brain tumors: clinical analysis of a series of 110 patients. Clin Neurol Neurosurg. 1996;98(2):171–5. https://doi.org/10.1016/0303-8467(96)00016-9. PMID: 8836593.

2. Katsuki M, Narita N, Sasaki K, Sato Y, Suzuki Y, Mashiyama S, Tominaga T. Standard values for temporal muscle thickness in the Japanese population who undergo brain check-up by magnetic resonance imaging. Surg Neurol Int. 2021;12:67. https://doi.org/10.25259/SNI_3_2021. PMID: 33767871; PMCID: PMC7982108.

3. Maslehaty H, Ngando H, Meila D, Brassel F, Scholz M, Petridis AK. Estimated low risk of rupture of small-sized unruptured intracranial aneurysms (UIAs) in relation to intracranial aneurysms in patients with subarachnoid haemorrhage. Acta Neurochir (Wien). 2013;155(6):1095–100; discussion 1100. https://doi.org/10.1007/s00701-013-1688-y. Epub 2013 Apr 5. PMID: 23558724.

4. Steiger HJ. Preventive neurosurgery: population-wide check-up examinations and correction of asymptomatic pathologies of the nervous system. Acta Neurochir (Wien). 2006;148(10):1075–83; discussion 1083. https://doi.org/10.1007/s00701-006-0882-6. Epub 2006 Sep 8. PMID: 16944049.

5. Wiebers DO, Piepgras DG, Meyer FB, Kallmes DF, Meissner I, Atkinson JL, Link MJ, Brown RD Jr. Pathogenesis, natural history, and treatment of unruptured intracranial aneurysms. Mayo Clin Proc. 2004;79(12):1572–83. https://doi.org/10.4065/79.12.1572. PMID: 15595346.

6. Williams LN, Brown RD Jr. Management of unruptured intracranial aneurysms. Neurol Clin Pract. 2013;3(2):99–108. https://doi.org/10.1212/CPJ.0b013e31828d9f6b. Erratum in: Neurol Clin Pract. 2014 Apr;4(2):98. PMID: 23914319; PMCID: PMC3721237.

7. Neyazi B, Sandalcioglu IE, Maslehaty H. Evaluation of the risk of rupture of intracranial aneurysms in patients with aneurysmal subarachnoid hemorrhage according to the PHASES score. Neurosurg Rev. 2019;42(2):489–92. https://doi.org/10.1007/s10143-018-0989-2. Epub 2018 Jun 11. PMID: 29948496.

8. Karhunen V, Bakker MK, Ruigrok YM, Gill D, Larsson SC. Modifiable risk factors for intracranial aneurysm and aneurysmal subarachnoid hemorrhage: a Mendelian randomization study. J Am Heart Assoc. 2021;10(22):e022277. https://doi.org/10.1161/JAHA.121.022277. Epub 2021 Nov 3. PMID: 34729997; PMCID: PMC8751955.

9. Teunissen LL, Rinkel GJ, Algra A, van Gijn J. Risk factors for subarachnoid hemorrhage: a systematic review. Stroke. 1996;27(3):544–9. https://doi.org/10.1161/01.str.27.3.544. PMID: 8610327.

10. Acosta JM, Cayron AF, Dupuy N, Pelli G, Foglia B, Haemmerli J, Allémann E, Bijlenga P, Kwak BR, Morel S. Effect of aneurysm and patient characteristics on intracranial aneurysm wall thickness. Front Cardiovasc Med. 2021;8:775307. https://doi.org/10.3389/fcvm.2021.775307. PMID: 34957259; PMCID: PMC8692777.

11. Giotta Lucifero A, Baldoncini M, Bruno N, Galzio R, Hernesniemi J, Luzzi S. Shedding the light on the natural history of intracranial aneurysms: an updated overview. Medicina (Kaunas). 2021;57(8):742. https://doi.org/10.3390/medicina57080742. PMID: 34440948; PMCID: PMC8400479.

12. Morel S, Bijlenga P, Kwak BR. Intracranial aneurysm wall (in)stability-current state of knowledge and clinical perspectives. Neurosurg Rev. 2022;45(2):1233–53. https://doi.org/10.1007/s10143-021-01672-5. Epub 2021 Nov 6. PMID: 34743248; PMCID: PMC8976821.

13. Perera R, Isoda H, Ishiguro K, Mizuno T, Takehara Y, Terada M, Tanoi C, Naito T, Sakahara H, Hiramatsu H, Namba H, Izumi T, Wakabayashi T, Kosugi T, Onishi Y, Alley M, Komori Y, Ikeda M, Naganawa S. Assessing the risk of intracranial aneurysm rupture using morphological and hemodynamic biomarkers evaluated from magnetic resonance fluid dynamics and computational fluid dynamics. Magn Reson Med Sci. 2020;19(4):333–44. https://doi.org/10.2463/mrms.mp.2019-0107. Epub 2020 Jan 17. PMID: 31956175; PMCID: PMC7809142.

14. Saqr KM, Rashad S, Tupin S, Niizuma K, Hassan T, Tominaga T, Ohta M. What does computational fluid dynamics tell us about intracranial aneurysms? A meta-analysis and critical review. J Cereb Blood Flow Metab. 2020;40(5):1021–39. https://doi.org/10.1177/0271678X19854640. Epub 2019 Jun 18. PMID: 31213162; PMCID: PMC7181089.

15. (a) Khan MO, Toro Arana V, Rubbert C, Cornelius JF, Fischer I, Bostelmann R, Mijderwijk HJ, Turowski B, Steiger HJ, May R, Petridis AK. Association between aneurysm hemodynamics and wall enhancement on 3D vessel wall MRI. J Neurosurg. 2020;134(2):565–75. (b) Petridis AK, Kaschner M, Cornelius JF, Kamp MA, Tortora A, Steiger HJ, Turowski B. A new imaging tool for realtime measurement of flow velocity in intracranial aneurysms. Clin Pract. 2017;7(3):975.

16. Molyneux AJ, Kerr RS, Yu LM, Clarke M, Sneade M, Yarnold JA, Sandercock P, International Subarachnoid Aneurysm Trial (ISAT) Collaborative Group. International subarachnoid aneurysm trial (ISAT) of neurosurgical clipping versus endovascular coiling in 2143 patients with ruptured intracranial aneurysms: a randomised comparison of effects on survival, dependency, seizures, rebleeding, subgroups, and aneurysm occlusion. Lancet. 2005;366:809–17.

17. Spetzler RF, McDougall CG, Albuquerque FC, Zabramski JM, Hills NK, Partovi S, Nakaji P, Wallace RC. The Barrow Ruptured Aneurysm Trial: 3-year results. J Neurosurg. 2013;119:146–57.

18. Spetzler RF, McDougall CG, Zabramski JM, Albuquerque FC, Hills NK, Nakaji P, Karis JP, Wallace RC. Ten-year analysis of saccular aneurysms in the Barrow Ruptured Aneurysm Trial. J Neurosurg. 2019;132:771–6.

19. Lee KS, Zhang JJY, Nguyen V, Han J, Johnson JN, Kirollos R, Teo M. The evolution of intracranial aneurysm treatment techniques and future directions. Neurosurg Rev. 2022;45(1):1–25. https://doi.org/10.1007/s10143-021-01543-z. Epub 2021 Apr 23. PMID: 33891216; PMCID: PMC8827391.

20. Dovey Z, Misra M, Thornton J, Charbel FT, Debrun GM, Ausman JI. Guglielmi detachable coiling for intracranial aneurysms: the story so far. Arch Neurol. 2001;58(4):559–64. https://doi.org/10.1001/archneur.58.4.559. PMID: 11295985.

21. Brilstra EH, Rinkel GJ. Treatment of ruptured intracranial aneurysms by embolization with controlled detachable coils. Neurologist. 2002;8:35–40.

22. Moret J, Cognard C, Weill A, Castaings L, Rey A. The "remodelling technique" in the treatment of wide neck intracranial aneurysms. Angiographic results and clinical follow-up in 56 cases. Interv Neuroradiol. 1997;3:21–35.

23. Zhao J, Lin H, Summers R, Yang M, Cousins BG, Tsui J. Current treatment strategies for intracranial aneurysms: an over- view. Angiology. 2018;69:17–30.

24. Gory B, Spiotta AM, Mangiafco S, Consoli A, Biondi A, Pomero E, Killer-Oberpfalzer M, Weber W, Riva R, Labeyrie PE, Turjman F. PulseRider stent-assisted coiling of wide-neck bifurcation aneurysms: periprocedural results in an international series. AJNR Am J Neuroradiol. 2016;37:130–5.

25. Phan K, Huo YR, Jia F, Phan S, Rao PJ, Mobbs RJ, Mortimer AM. Meta-analysis of stent-assisted coiling versus coiling-only for the treatment of intracranial aneurysms. J Clin Neurosci. 2016;31:15–22.

26. Pranata R, Yonas E, Vania R, Sidipratomo P, July J. Efficacy and safety of PulseRider for treatment of wide-necked intracranial aneurysm—a systematic review and meta-analysis. Interv Neuroradiol. 2021;27:60–7.

27. Sorenson TJ, Iacobucci M, Murad MH, Spelle L, Moret J, Lanzino G. The pCONUS bifurcation aneurysm implants for endovascular treatment of adults with intracranial aneurysms: a systematic review and meta-analysis. Surg Neurol Int. 2019;10:24.

28. Baxter BW, Rosso D, Lownie SP. Double microcatheter technique for detachable coil treatment of large, wide-necked intracranial aneurysms. AJNR Am J Neuroradiol. 1998;19:1176–8.

29. Kwon OK, Kim SH, Kwon BJ, Kang HS, Kim JH, Oh CW, Han MH. Endovascular treatment of wide-necked aneurysms by using two microcatheters: techniques and outcomes in 25 patients. AJNR Am J Neuroradiol. 2005;26:894–900.

30. Shin YS, Kim DI, Lee SI, Chung JI, Yoon PH, Lee KC. The usefulness of the new "double-catheter technique" in the treatment of parent artery incorporated wide-necked aneurysm with guglielmi detachable coils. Technical notes. Interv Neuroradiol. 2000;6:61–4.

31. Yin L, Wei M, Ren H. Double microcatheter technique for coil embolization of small aneurysms with unfavorable configurations: a comparative study of the aneurysms that are ≤3 mm or >3 mm. Interv Neuroradiol. 2016;22:158–64.

32. Zhao J, Lin H, Summers R, Yang M, Cousins BG, Tsui J. Current treatment strategies for intracranial aneurysms: an overview. Angiology. 2018;69:17–30.

33. Madaelil TP, Moran CJ, Cross DT, Kansagra AP. Flow diversion in ruptured intracranial aneurysms: a meta-analysis. AJNR Am J Neuroradiol. 2017;38:590–5.

34. Zhang M, Anzai H, Chopard B, Ohta M. Towards the patient-specific design of flow diverters made from helix-like wires: an optimization study. Biomed Eng Online. 2016;15:159.

35. Cras TY, Bos D, Ikram MA, Vergouwen MDI, Dippel DWJ, Voortman T, Adams HHH, Vernooij MW, Roozenbeek B. Determinants of the presence and size of intracranial aneurysms in the general population: the Rotterdam Study. Stroke. 2020;51(7):2103–10. https://doi.org/10.1161/STROKEAHA.120.029296. Epub 2020 Jun 10. PMID: 32517578; PMCID: PMC7306261.

36. Pontes FGB, da Silva EM, Baptista-Silva JC, Vasconcelos V. Treatments for unruptured intracranial aneurysms. Cochrane Database Syst Rev. 2021;5(5):CD013312. https://doi.org/10.1002/14651858.CD013312.pub2. PMID: 33971026; PMCID: PMC8109849.

37. Vlak MH, Algra A, Brandenburg R, Rinkel GJ. Prevalence of unruptured intracranial aneurysms, with emphasis on sex, age, comorbidity, country, and time period: a systematic review and meta-analysis. Lancet Neurol. 2011;10(7):626–36. https://doi.org/10.1016/S1474-4422(11)70109-0. PMID: 21641282.

38. Bakker MK, van der Spek RAA, van Rheenen W, Morel S, Bourcier R, Hostettler IC, Alg VS, van Eijk KR, Koido M, Akiyama M, Terao C, Matsuda K, Walters RG, Lin K, Li L, Millwood IY, Chen Z, Rouleau GA, Zhou S, Rannikmäe K, Sudlow CLM, Houlden H, van den Berg LH, Dina C, Naggara O, Gentric JC, Shotar E, Eugene F, Desal H, Winsvold BS, Borte S, Johnsen MB, Brumpton BM, Sandvei MS, Willer CJ, Hveem K, Zwart JA, Verschuren WMM, Friedrich CM, Hirsch S, Schilling S, Dauvillier J, Martin O; HUNT All-In Stroke; China Kadoorie Biobank Collaborative Group; BioBank Japan Project Consortium; ICAN Study Group; CADISP Group; Genetics and Observational Subarachnoid Haemorrhage (GOSH) Study investigators; International Stroke Genetics Consortium (ISGC); Jones GT, Bown MJ, Ko NU, Kim H, Coleman JRI, Breen G, Zaroff JG, Klijn CJM, Malik R, Dichgans M, Sargurupremraj M, Tatlisumak T, Amouyel P, Debette S, Rinkel GJE, Worrall BB, Pera J, Slowik A, Gaál-Paavola EI, Niemelä M, Jääskeläinen JE, von Und Zu Fraunberg M, Lindgren A, Broderick JP, Werring DJ, Woo D, Redon R, Bijlenga P, Kamatani Y, Veldink JH, Ruigrok YM. Genome-wide association study of intracranial aneurysms identifies 17 risk loci and genetic overlap with clinical risk factors. Nat Genet. 2020;52(12):1303–13. https://doi.org/10.1038/s41588-020-00725-7. Epub 2020 Nov 16. Erratum in: Nat Genet. 2020 Dec 22; PMID: 33199917; PMCID: PMC7116530.

39. Dewan MC, Rattani A, Fieggen G, Arraez MA, Servadei F, Boop FA, Johnson WD, Warf BC, Park KB. Global neurosurgery: the current capacity and deficit in the provision of essential neurosurgical care. Executive Summary of the Global Neurosurgery Initiative at the Program in Global Surgery and Social Change. J Neurosurg. 2018;130(4):1055–64. https://doi.org/10.3171/2017.11.JNS171500. PMID: 29701548.

40. Tetinou F, Kanmounye US, Nitcheu I, Ndajiwo AB, Bankole NDA. P120 The burden of the management of cerebral aneurysms in Africa: a scoping review. BJS Open. 2021;5(Suppl 1):zrab032.119. https://doi.org/10.1093/bjsopen/zrab032.119. PMCID: PMC8153800.

41. Lawton MT. Seven bypasses: tenets and techniques for revascularization. New York: Thieme Medical Publishers, Inc.; 2018. p. 150–62.

42. Petridis AK, Kinzel A, Schreiber L, Parvin R, Scholz M, Maslehaty H. Procedural paradigm in intraoperative aneurysm clipping with microdoppler ultrasound, near-infrared indocyanine green videoangiography and intraoperative angiography. J Neurol Disord. 2014;2:3.

43. Vourla E, Filis A, Cornelius JF, Bostelmann R, Turowski B, Kalakoti P, Rubbert C, Suresh MP, Tortora A, Steiger HJ, Petridis AK. Natural history of de novo aneurysm formation in patients with treated aneurysmatic subarachnoid hemorrhage: a ten-year follow-up. World Neurosurg. 2019;122:e291–5. https://doi.org/10.1016/j.wneu.2018.10.022. Epub 2018 Oct 12. PMID: 30321678.

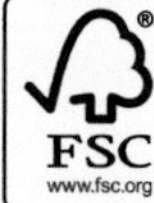